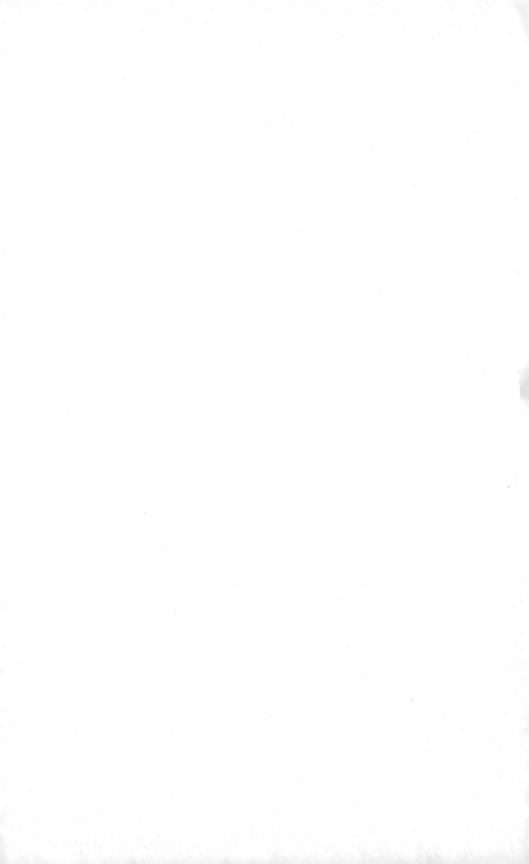

Cambridge Elements ≡

Elements in Genetics in Epilepsy
edited by
Annapurna H. Poduri
Boston Children's Hospital and Harvard Medical School
Alfred L. George, Jr.
Northwestern University Feinberg School of Medicine
Erin L. Heinzen
University of North Carolina, Chapel Hill
Sara James
KCNQ2 Cure Alliance and Genetic Epilepsy Team Australia

SCN2A-RELATED DISORDERS

Edited by

Alfred L. George, Jr.
*Northwestern University Feinberg
School of Medicine*

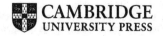

CAMBRIDGE
UNIVERSITY PRESS

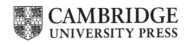

CAMBRIDGE
UNIVERSITY PRESS

Shaftesbury Road, Cambridge CB2 8EA, United Kingdom

One Liberty Plaza, 20th Floor, New York, NY 10006, USA

477 Williamstown Road, Port Melbourne, VIC 3207, Australia

314–321, 3rd Floor, Plot 3, Splendor Forum, Jasola District Centre,
New Delhi – 110025, India

103 Penang Road, #05–06/07, Visioncrest Commercial, Singapore 238467

Cambridge University Press is part of Cambridge University Press & Assessment,
a department of the University of Cambridge.

We share the University's mission to contribute to society through the pursuit of education,
learning and research at the highest international levels of excellence.

www.cambridge.org
Information on this title: www.cambridge.org/9781009530330
DOI: 10.1017/9781009530361

First published 2024

A catalogue record for this publication is available from the British Library.

ISBN 978-1-009-53033-0 Hardback
ISBN 978-1-009-53037-8 Paperback
ISSN 2633-2086 (online)
ISSN 2633-2078 (print)

Additional resources for this publication at http://www.cambridge.org/scn2a

Cambridge University Press & Assessment has no responsibility for the persistence
or accuracy of URLs for external or third-party internet websites referred to in this
publication and does not guarantee that any content on such websites is, or will
remain, accurate or appropriate.

Every effort has been made in preparing this Element to provide accurate and up-to-date
information which is in accord with accepted standards and practice at the time of publication.
Although case histories are drawn from actual cases, every effort has been made to disguise the
identities of the individuals involved. Nevertheless, the authors, editors and publishers can make
no warranties that the information contained herein is totally free from error, not least because
clinical standards are constantly changing through research and regulation. The authors, editors
and publishers therefore disclaim all liability for direct or consequential damages resulting from
the use of material contained in this Element. Readers are strongly advised to pay careful attention
to information provided by the manufacturer of any drugs or equipment that they plan to use.

SCN2A-Related Disorders

Elements in Genetics in Epilepsy

DOI: 10.1017/9781009530361
First published online: November 2024

Edited by Alfred L. George, Jr.
Northwestern University Feinberg School of Medicine

Editor for correspondence: Alfred L. George Jr., al.george@northwestern.edu

Abstract: *SCN2A* encodes a voltage-gated sodium channel (designated $Na_V1.2$) vital for generating neuronal action potentials (APs). Pathogenic *SCN2A* variants are associated with a diverse array of neurodevelopmental disorders featuring neonatal or infantile onset epilepsy, developmental delay, autism, intellectual disability, and movement disorders. This remarkable clinical heterogeneity is mirrored by extensive allelic heterogeneity and complex genotype–phenotype relationships partially explained by divergent functional consequences of pathogenic variants. Emerging therapeutic strategies targeted to specific patterns of $Na_V1.2$ dysfunction offer hope for improving the lives of individuals affected by *SCN2A*-related disorders. This Element provides a review of the clinical features, genetic basis, pathophysiology, pharmacology, and treatment of these genetic conditions authored by leading experts in the field and accompanied by perspectives shared by affected families. This title is also available as Open Access on Cambridge Core.

Keywords: sodium channel, epilepsy, epileptic encephalopathy, neonatal seizures, epilepsy genetics, autism spectrum disorder, neurodevelopmental disorder, intellectual disability, precision medicine

ISBNs: 9781009530330 (HB), 9781009530378 (PB), 9781009530361 (OC)
ISSNs: 2633-2086 (online), 2633-2078 (print)

Contents

Contributors

Megan Abbott
University of Colorado School of Medicine
Kevin J. Bender
University of California, San Francisco
Andreas Brunklaus
Royal Hospital for Children and University of Glasgow
Scott Demarest
University of Colorado School of Medicine
Shawn Egan
FamilieSCN2A Foundation
Isabel Haviland
Boston Children's Hospital and Harvard Medical School
Jennifer A. Kearney
Northwestern University Feinberg School of Medicine
Leah Schust Myers
FamilieSCN2A Foundation
Heather E. Olson
Boston Children's Hospital and Harvard Medical School
Stephan J. Sanders
University of Oxford
Christina SanInocencio
FamilieSCN2A Foundation
Joseph Symonds
Royal Hospital for Children and University of Glasgow
Christopher H. Thompson
Northwestern University Feinberg School of Medicine

Introduction

This is the second gene-focused Element of the Cambridge Elements series on Genetics in Epilepsy launched in September 2021 [1]. The goal of this Element is to provide an in-depth, state-of-the-art review of clinical, genetic, basic science, and family perspectives on neurological and neurodevelopmental disorders (NDD) associated with pathogenic variants in *SCN2A*, which encodes a major voltage-gated sodium ion channel (designated Na$_V$1.2) in the brain. The *SCN2A*-related disorders are clinically heterogenous with features ranging from neonatal and infantile onset epilepsy, late onset epileptic encephalopathy, autism spectrum disorder (ASD), and intellectual disability (ID). In addition to phenotype diversity, the widespread use of clinical genetic testing has resulted in more than 1,000 *SCN2A* variants deposited in ClinVar. With the explosion in genetic variant identification has come recognition of genotype–phenotype relationships, which when coupled with experimental demonstration of functional perturbations are guiding new therapeutic approaches. Investigations into the biology of *SCN2A* has led to fundamental discoveries about the physiology and pathophysiology of synaptic connections and neural circuits. As one of the earliest known epilepsy genes, *SCN2A* has emerged as an important genetic factor in neurodevelopment and NDD.

We hope this Element will provide opportunities for families, trainees, and health care professionals to learn about *SCN2A*-related disorders. Subsections of this Element offer complete discussions about clinical features, pathophysiology, genetics, model systems, and treatment. This Element begins with perspectives from parents and caregivers of children with these disorders, made possible by a parent-led advocacy group (the FamilieSCN2A Foundation). The following subsections are devoted to clinical features, genotype–phenotype correlations, basic science, and current and future therapeutic approaches. Thus, this Element on *SCN2A*-related disorders provides a comprehensive and in-depth review of the state of knowledge in this field, which should be valuable to scientists, clinicians, trainees, and families interested in the topic.

In addition to a thorough and informative narrative, this Element is augmented by video content, including interviews with parents of children with *SCN2A*-related disorders (Video 1); with Dr. Matthew State (Professor and Chair, Department of Psychiatry and Behavioral Sciences, University of California, San Francisco) on the genomics of ASD and the discovery of *SCN2A* as a major risk factor (Video 2); and with Dr. Steven Petrou (Professor of Neuroscience, University of Melbourne, and Chief Scientific Officer at Praxis Precision Medicines) on his career evolution from academic research to a new pharmaceutical company specializing in precision medicine for rare neurological diseases (Video 3).

This was a team effort that we hope provides inspiration to future clinicians, researchers, and patient advocates. We hope you enjoy learning about this important epilepsy gene.

Patient, Family, and Foundation Perspectives

Pathogenic variants in the *SCN2A* gene are associated with a broad spectrum of complex NDD that are collectively designated as *SCN2A*-related disorders. The primary clinical manifestations include epilepsy, ASD, movement disorders, and ID. The severity of these conditions varies among individuals, ranging from mild and well controlled to severe and treatment resistant. Even individuals with mild clinical phenotypes exhibit significant impairments compared to their age-matched peers. Those on the severe end of the spectrum are profoundly affected and heavily reliant on their caregivers for all aspects of daily life. Given the complexity of *SCN2A*-related disorders, clinical care teams are often multi-disciplinary, emphasizing the importance of coordinated efforts to optimize care and minimize clinical risks (Figure 1).

FamilieSCN2A Foundation

The FamilieSCN2A Foundation, founded in 2015, is the largest nonprofit patient advocacy organization representing *SCN2A*-related disorders and has the broadest international footprint among other *SCN2A* patient-advocacy groups. Focused on creating an engaged ecosystem, FamilieSCN2A Foundation acts as a central

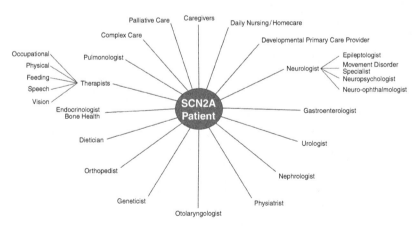

Figure 1 Diagram of multispecialty care of a patient with an *SCN2A*-related disorder.

liaison between patients, caregivers, scientists, clinicians, and industry. They also work in close partnership with other large foundations such as the Simons Foundation and the Chan Zuckerberg Initiative. "Families" is part of the Foundation's name because these rare and devastating conditions affect the entire family. The Foundation strives every day and, in every way, to improve the lives of not only the patients but also the entire family.

The missions of the Foundation are to accelerate research, foster a sense of community, and advocate for improvements in the lives of those affected. The Foundation's vision is centered around achieving effective treatments and cures for all *SCN2A*-related disorders. The core values of the Foundation are urgency, integrity, collaboration, and inclusion. FamilieSCN2A strives to provide families and professionals with the information and tools needed for a rapid and accurate diagnosis as well as the resources needed to tailor treatments based on the patients' and families' goals informed by research knowledge.

Before 2014, there was little hope for children or families diagnosed with an *SCN2A*-related disorder. There were no specialists treating the condition, no support groups for families desperately seeking answers, and no researchers investigating cures. This void created a gravity that pulled together a small group of thoughtful, committed parents who sought to build a better world for their children, and thus the FamilieSCN2A Foundation was born. The Foundation grew quickly as other parents and professionals were inspired and empowered by the stated vision: a world with effective treatments and cures for all *SCN2A*-related disorders. As momentum built, the Foundation attracted board members that shared the core values and missions. A timeline of Foundation milestones is presented in Figure 2.

Advocacy is critical to the mission of FamilieSCN2A. The tenets of their advocacy strategy are: awareness, empowerment, evidence-based research, and equity. Successful advocacy requires awareness within the patient/family community and beyond. Awareness of *SCN2A*-related disorders began with the first online support group using the Facebook platform, which launched in 2013 with just five members. Today, there are more than 1,000 participants. This private, robust group is a safe space for families, patients, and caregivers to share their journey, ask questions, learn from one another, and reduce feelings of isolation. The community of patient caregivers remains a pillar of support for individuals affected by *SCN2A*-related disorders.

To extend awareness beyond families, the FamilieSCN2A Foundation spearheads various awareness initiatives including state proclamations, listening sessions with the Food and Drug Administration (FDA), providing information to policymakers and drug developers, and organizing caregiver testimonies that are intended to raise

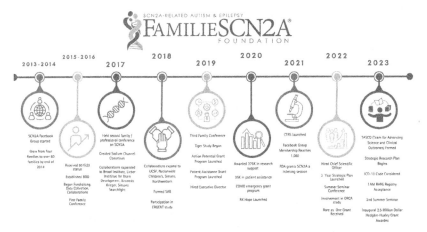

Figure 2 Timeline of major events involving the FamilieSCN2A Foundation.

awareness of the burden of disease. Education, which is vital for a community actively engaged in collaboration with clinicians, scientists, and industry, has been an important Foundation strategy. As such, the FamilieSCN2A Foundation organizes an annual family and professional conference that leaves participants feeling empowered, educated, and hopeful. Supplementing the educational initiatives are programs that support families both emotionally and financially. Initiatives include Family Meet Up Grants, a Birthday Club, and a Patient Assistance Grant program that has awarded more than $65,000 to families since 2015.

The accomplishments of the FamilieSCN2A Foundation include $4 million raised since 2015, 1,200 families supported globally, strategic partnerships with leading academic researchers, a voice with the FDA, representation at international conferences, and a growing attendance at the annual family and professional symposium. Its founders, board members, volunteers, and community (including researchers and clinicians) together have made significant progress in a thoughtful way and committed to changing the world for those affected with *SCN2A*-related disorders.

Family and Caregiver Perspectives

There is a dearth of literature that describes the burden of care and health-related quality of life (HRQoL) as they relate to *SCN2A*-related disorders. While Cohen and colleagues [2] summarized quality of life and its determinants in developmental and epileptic encephalopathies (DEEs), for which *SCN2A* pathogenic variants accounted for 24 percent of the cases (n=42/173), no peer-reviewed HRQoL studies have been published specific to *SCN2A*-related disorders. Given the severity of *SCN2A*-related disorders and their impact on individuals and their families, it is imperative that additional HRQoL studies be conducted. Further, understanding the lived experiences of patients and their caregivers facing rare neurologic diseases is critical to advancing patient-centered outcomes research and informing clinical trial design. Lived experiences also highlight unmet needs of the *SCN2A*-related disorders community and describe the nuances of the disease beyond clinical care. Thus, this section provides a glimpse into some of the challenges families face on a daily basis and illustrates why the patient voice is a fundamental component that complements the clinical and scientific literature on *SCN2A*-related disorders.

To capture the family perspective, the FamilieSCN2A Foundation interviewed caregivers of individuals with *SCN2A*-related disorders. Interviews were transcribed and edited into a short video that highlights various aspects of the disorder (Video 1).

> *I felt shattered and heartbroken. The doctors did not know anything about this diagnosis. They were new to it but luckily, they did give us all the information of the FamilieSCN2A foundation. That was helpful.*
>
> — Sofia's mom, United States

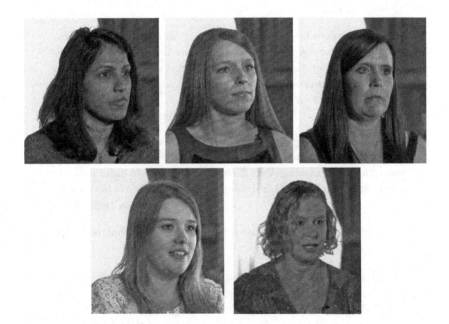

Video 1 Parents (Sandya Crasta, Liz Hendrickx, Amy Richards, Ashley Taylor, Tracy Umezu) discussing experiences caring for their children with *SCN2A*-related disorders.

A transcript of this video is available in the Appendix. The video file is available at www.cambridge.org/scn2a

In addition, the following paraphrased quotes describe how families felt when they received a diagnosis of *SCN2A*-related disorders.

Terrible. My world just fell apart. I didn't know what to do. Didn't know where to look because in Belgium, there just aren't many cases. The doctors told me not to Google it, and that was pretty scary.

– Charlie's mom, Belgium

I felt a mixture of emotions for the first 23 months of my son's life. He was initially neurotypical, then seizures started. Within two months of seizures starting, we got the diagnosis. I felt overwhelmed. There was a little bit of excitement knowing that there's something that they can possibly treat, but at the same time scary that they knew very little about it. I was scared for the future.

– Hudson's mom, United States

I was actually thrilled. It was such a relief to finally figure out what was wrong. I knew from infancy that something was wrong. I always equated it to a juggling act: she has GI reflux, and she's got a tic-like behavior, and she's got apraxia of speech, and she has double hip dysplasia. I kept asking, so then what is it? There has to be something underlying. I just wanted a name for it.

– Erin's mom, United States

The following express the difficulties of having a child affected with a *SCN2A*-related disorder.

Charlotte was born having over 400 seizures a day and she was very prone to illness. As her life went on, she had more and more seizures, and towards the end of her life, she was in status most of the time and her brain wasn't functioning anymore. The hardest part for me was that I am an Intensive Care Unit nurse and knew too much.

– Charlotte's mom, United States

It's kind of like stripping everything away that I had envisioned for my child. I had to re-evaluate what his future might look like. I watched him suffer and was not able to do anything about it. He still pushes through with a smile, but it's challenging to know that there's nothing I can do about it at this moment.

– Hudson's mom, United States

The way families feel about a cure for *SCN2A*-related disorders is expressed by these statements.

I believe in a cure. There are a lot of prayers as well as just the parental force of the FamilieSCN2A foundation that have come together to make me feel hopeful that there would someday be a cure.

– Sofia's mom, United States

I always believe in a cure. That's the main reason why I attend the conferences. That why we're not giving up, why we're going across the globe to find people who understand and who are willing to work with us. That's why I'm screaming from the rooftops telling everyone, "this is what my child has!" I tell every cab driver. I'm here for this, this is my daughter, she has this, I'm telling everyone.

– Charlie's mom, Belgium

I think there's going to be a cure. I'm not 100 percent sure it's going to be in her lifetime.

– Erin's mom, United States

These quotes were in response to asking parents how they have been impacted by FamilieSCN2A Foundation.

We ask questions and we get answers that we don't get from our doctors. We get mental as well as emotional support from each other, even coming to the conferences and learning about what the research is done or just meeting other families has been possible through the funding that is available through the FamilieSCN2A Foundation for which I am very grateful.

– Sophia's mom, United States

It's a huge support system knowing that I'm not alone and that there are others that understand my struggle. It's a judgment-free zone. It's a source of hope because I see what the foundation is doing. It gives me hope that people care and they are trying to do something about SCN2A.

– Hudson's mom, United States

I believe that the foundation provides a community of support for our families. It gives families hope and I am really excited at the research that they initiated, to get doctors excited about researching this disease, and putting money towards finding a cure or at least a better quality of life for our kids.

– Charlotte's mom, United States

In an effort to build upon the interview data, FamilieSCN2A disseminated a questionnaire to their community in March 2023 that asked questions related to the consequences of caregiving. Two specific questions generated data that formed visual representations of (1) how caregivers felt when their children were first diagnosed and (2) what they wished their providers knew about *SCN2A*-related disorders. Figure 3 illustrates word clouds representing these responses.

Given the dearth of literature describing the challenges and consequences of caring for *SCN2A*-related disorders for patients and their families, combined with the speed at which *SCN2A*-related disorders are being studied and the simultaneous growth of the FamilieSCN2A Foundation, we hope this section has provided a thorough overview that highlights various aspects of the disorder and leaves families feeling empowered and health care professionals with valuable insights to navigate the complexities associated with *SCN2A*-related disorders.

Clinical Spectrum and Genotype–Phenotype Correlations

Pathogenic *SCN2A* variants are associated with a range of NDD with or without epilepsy, having symptom onset anytime between the first day of life through later childhood (Figure 4). Due to the variability in clinical presentation, data on

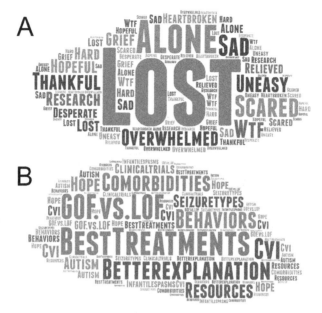

Figure 3 Word clouds generated from caregiver responses. (A) Responses expressing how caregivers felt when their child was first diagnosed. (B) Responses expressing what caregivers wished their health care providers knew about *SCN2A*-related disorders.

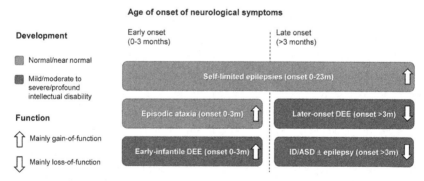

Figure 4 Clinical spectrum of *SCN2A*-related disorders. Black-shaded boxes indicate phenotypes associated with normal development. Unshaded boxes indicate phenotypes associated with mild or moderate to severe or profound ID. Arrows indicate predominant associated functional effects of *SCN2A* variants in each condition. Typical age of onset is given in months (m) and generally refers to the onset of seizures.

the incidence of *SCN2A*-related disorders is not complete. For example, epilepsy patient cohorts exclude cases of NDD that do not have seizures. Expanded genetic testing that includes a wider spectrum of NDD will likely reveal an even greater genotype and phenotype diversity.

In a meta-analysis of genetic findings discovered using next generation sequencing-based gene panels, *SCN2A* was the fourth most commonly implicated gene in monogenic epilepsy (after *SCN1A*, *KCNQ2*, and *CDKL5*) accounting for 7 percent of cases [3]. By comparison, *SCN1A*-associated epilepsy accounted for nearly three times as many cases (19 percent). The incidence of *SCN1A*-associated epilepsy was accurately estimated as 1 per 12,200 live births from a population-based cohort study in Scotland [4]. Based on the assumption that *SCN1A*-associated epilepsy is approximately three times more common than *SCN2A*-associated epilepsy, one might expect the incidence of *SCN2A*-related epilepsy to be in the range of 1 in 30,000 to 50,000 live births. An estimate of 1 per 78,608 live births for *SCN2A*-related epilepsy was based previously on observing seven cases of *SCN2A*-related epilepsy diagnosed in the single national Danish testing center between 2006 and 2014 [5].

A comparable incidence estimate of *SCN2A*-related NDD comes from the UK Deciphering Developmental Disorders (DDD) study [6,7], a national multicenter study in which participants with a wide range of developmental disorders underwent whole exome sequencing (WES). The DDD incidence estimate includes *SCN2A*-related NDD without epilepsy as a feature, but excludes self-limited and familial epilepsy cases. Analyzing the first 4,293 families in the DDD study, the authors estimated that 42 percent of the cohort carried a disease-causing de novo variant in any gene. They further estimated that a de novo variant can be expected to result in a developmental disorder between 1 in 213–448 births. Because 19 study participants with *SCN2A*-related NDD were among these 4,293 families, the incidence of *SCN2A*-related NDD can be estimated as 1 per 47,000 to 100,000 live births.

Nearly all individuals with *SCN2A* variants develop epilepsy at some point in their life. It is estimated that about half of individuals with *SCN2A*-related NDD will present with seizures in the neonatal period [5,8], and 80 percent will develop seizures within the first six months of life [5,8]. Focal seizures are the most common seizure type, reported in 90 percent of individuals, and epileptic spasms occur in up to 50 percent of individuals with *SCN2A*-related NDD [8]. Nearly 80 percent of individuals with *SCN2A*-related epilepsy have comorbid developmental delay [8]. Mosaicism is estimated to occur in 6.4 percent of pathogenic *SCN2A* variants, present at only 11.6 percent of variant reads (range: 11.6–39.5 percent) [9].

Self-limited Epilepsies

Self-limited familial neonatal-infantile epilepsy (SeLFNIE), previously known as benign familial neonatal-infantile epilepsy, was the first reported *SCN2A*-related disorder [10,11]. Self-limited epilepsies represent approximately 20 percent of the phenotypic spectrum of reported *SCN2A*-related disorders [12], and include neonatal, neonatal-infantile, and infantile subtypes, which are classified by age of seizure onset along with family history [13]. Seizure onset ranges from 2 days to 23 months with a mean of 11.2 ± 9.2 weeks and median of 13 weeks [11,12]. Approximately half of affected individuals have onset before age one month [5]. Seizures are typically focal with head and eye deviation along with tonic or clonic features and possibly apnea; some evolve to bilateral tonic-clonic seizures [10,11,14,15]. Seizures may occur in brief clusters (20 seconds to 3 minutes), are most often afebrile, and are usually controlled with single antiseizure medications such as phenobarbital, phenytoin, oxcarbazepine, clobazam, zonisamide, or valproic acid [5,8,11,14]. Electroencephalograms are generally normal or show focal epileptiform activity without severe encephalopathy patterns, and seizures typically resolve by age 12 months with rare recurrence later in life [5,8,11,14]. Developmental milestones and cognitive outcomes are typically normal, and *SCN2A* variants in SeLFNIE are frequently inherited with high penetrance. Distinguishing SeLFNIE from more severe DEEs at the time of seizure onset can be challenging. A representative clinical scenario is described in Box 1.

Box 1 A three-week-old infant presented with focal motor, evolving to bilateral tonic-clonic, seizures. He had been born at term with no prenatal or perinatal complications. Interictal encephalography (EEG) demonstrated normal background rhythms. Seizures were controlled with carbamazepine. He was weaned off antiseizure medication at two years. He had recurrence of a single generalized tonic-clonic seizure following a concussion at six years but had a normal 24-hour EEG. Cognitive and developmental outcome was normal at six years.

The primary differential diagnoses for SeLFNIE, assuming structural brain imaging is normal or demonstrates nonspecific changes, include the following:

➤ *KCNQ2*-related epilepsy: This condition presents with a range from self-limited infantile epilepsy to DEE with or without burst suppression on electroencephalography (EEG). The seizure onset is more often neonatal and responds well to carbamazepine or other sodium channel blockers [11,16,17].

➢ *PRRT2*-related epilepsy: This disorder is characterized by self-limited infant-ile epilepsy with focal motor seizures and an excellent response to antiseizure medication, particularly sodium channel blockers [18,19]. Seizure onset is typically at age 4–12 months with resolution by two years. Paroxysmal kinesigenic dyskinesia is also associated with pathogenic *PRRT2* variants but symptoms may start after seizure onset [19,20,21].

➢ *SCN8A*-related epilepsy: Epilepsy associated with pathogenic *SCN8A* variants can manifest as self-limited infantile epilepsy or DEE. Median age of onset is approximately six months. Seizure types include focal, multifocal, or bilateral tonic-clonic. In the DEE phenotype, epileptic spasms are reported. Seizures in DEE caused by gain-of-function (GOF) *SCN8A* variants are reported to respond favorably to sodium channel blockers, though high doses are often required [22]. Movement disorders including myoclonus, tremor, and paroxysmal dyskinesias are reported [23,24,26].

Early Infantile Developmental and Epileptic Encephalopathy

DEE represents the most frequent clinical presentation among published cases of *SCN2A*-related disorders. The early infantile subtype of DEE is characterized by epilepsy onset within the first three months of life, usually in the neonatal period, and represented 36 percent of participants in a study of 201 individuals with *SCN2A*-related disorders [5]. In this study, 43 percent (31 of 71) of the early infantile DEE subset had an identifiable epilepsy syndrome, including early infantile DEE with burst suppression on EEG (18 of 71) and epilepsy of infancy with migrating focal seizures (EIMFS) (13 of 71), while the remaining 56 percent (40 of 71) had unclassifiable epilepsies with focal or generalized seizure types including tonic, tonic-clonic, and epileptic spasms. Initial inter-ictal EEG often shows a burst-suppression pattern or multifocal spikes [5,27,28].

Intellectual disability, often profound or severe, is present in a majority of individuals. Comorbid movement disorders are common, including dystonia, chorea, choreoathetosis, and dyskinesia [5,28,29]. Other reported comorbidities include cortical visual impairment, microcephaly, and features of dysautonomia such as temperature instability (hypo- or hyperthermia) and tachycardia [5,28,29]. Brain MRI may be normal or show cerebral atrophy, hypomyelina-tion, and T2 hyperintensities, among other abnormalities [5,27,29,30]. These MRI findings are nonspecific, and cerebral atrophy specifically has been asso-ciated with other causes of early infantile developmental encephalopathy [13,27]. Rare individuals with *SCN2A*-related DEE have been found to have polymicrogyria [31,32,33], suggesting a potential role of sodium channels in neuronal migration during brain development. A representative clinical scenario is described in Box 2.

Specific early infantile DEE phenotypes associated with pathogenic *SCN2A* variants are described next.

Box 2 *A female infant presented on day one of life with multiple predominantly focal tonic seizures per day. EEG initially showed burst suppression evolving to generalized slowing with multifocal or bi-frontal epileptiform activity. Phenytoin was the most effective antiseizure medication but did not achieve seizure freedom. Oxcarbazepine treatment was associated with a partial response and greater alertness but was accompanied by hyponatremia. A combination of lacosamide and lamotrigine resulted in two years of near seizure-freedom, with breakthrough only in the setting of missed or late doses. A likely pathogenic, de novo variant in SCN2A was identified by epilepsy gene panel testing.*

At nine years of age, the patient exhibited global developmental delay with axial hypotonia and was unable to sit independently. She showed no purposeful hand use, smiled in response to voices but expressive communication was limited to nonspecific vocalizations. She had cortical visual impairment and made limited eye contact. Other medical issues included mild scoliosis, oral phase dysphagia with poor weight gain, and irritability.

Epilepsy of Infancy with Migrating Focal Seizures (EIMFS)

EIMFS is characterized by multiple types of focal seizures that "migrate" from one hemisphere to the other, usually accompanied by severe developmental impairment [29]. *SCN2A* is second to *KCNT1* as the most frequently identified gene in EIMFS [28,29]. In these two cited studies of individuals with EIMFS and *SCN2A* variants (22 total), onset of seizures occurred between the first day of life and eight weeks for most (20/22), and less commonly after age one year (2/22). All had multifocal spikes on EEG.

Early Infantile DEE with Burst Suppression

SCN2A has been identified as a common gene associated with early infantile DEE with burst suppression on EEG formerly called Ohtahara syndrome [8,27,29,30,31,34,35]. Seizure types typically include epileptic spasms, tonic seizures, and/or myoclonic seizures [13,36]. In two studies of individuals with early infantile DEE, *SCN2A* variants were identified in 9/67 (13.4 percent) and

2/33 (7 percent) respectively [27,34]. Infantile epileptic spasms syndrome (IESS) has also been reported in individuals with *SCN2A*-related early infantile DEE, either independently or evolving from an initial presentation as early infantile DEE with burst suppression [8].

Prognosis is variable. With regard to epilepsy, response to sodium channel blocking antiseizure medications in *SCN2A*-related early infantile DEE is often favorable, but high doses are often needed and there are reports of seizure relapse when plasma drug levels drop below a certain threshold [5,29]. There have been several reported instances of sudden unexpected death in epilepsy (SUDEP) in this subset of individuals [5,8,29], which warrants consideration in discussing the prognosis with families. Other reported causes of early death include pneumonia (age 21 months) [29], respiratory failure during treatment of pneumonia [30], iatrogenic cardiorespiratory failure (age 19 days) [37], severe infection, and status epilepticus [5].

The primary differential diagnoses for this group, assuming structural brain imaging is normal or demonstrates nonspecific changes, include the following:

> *KCNT1*-related disorder: As mentioned previously, *KCNT1* is the gene most frequently associated with EIMFS [28,29]. Differentiating features that are more associated with *SCN2A* include presence of severe movement disorders and seizure response to phenytoin [29,38]. Age of seizure onset may also be slightly later in those with *KCNT1*-associated EIMFS (median 3.5 weeks, compared to median of 3.5 days in those with *SCN2A*-associated EIMFS) [28]. Prognosis appears to be less favorable in *KCNT1*-related EIMFS, with higher reported rates of severe to profound developmental impairment, refractory epilepsy, and SUDEP compared to those with *SCN2A* variants [5,28,39].

> *KCNQ2*-related disorder: Variants in *KCNQ2* are a frequently discovered genetic cause of early infantile DEE with burst suppression [27,40], and should be considered in the differential diagnosis of a patient with this phenotype. Neonatal onset seizures associated with pathogenic *KCNQ2* variant are also responsive to sodium channel blocking antiseizure medications [17], which may resemble the response of individuals with *SCN2A* GOF variants.

Later Onset Developmental and Epileptic Encephalopathies

DEEs presenting after three months of age constitute the second largest group (20–30 percent) with pathogenic *SCN2A* variants [5,41]. Affected individuals typically present with generalized tonic-clonic, absence, and myoclonic seizures along with EEG features of generalized spike and wave or multifocal spikes. A number of distinct epilepsy syndrome presentations in this later onset group have been described. This includes individuals with IESS evolving to Lennox-Gastaut syndrome (LGS), myoclonic atonic epilepsy (MAE), and focal epilepsies with a condition resembling electrical status epilepticus during slow-wave sleep (ESES). Brain imaging is mostly normal with the exception of occasional nonspecific cortical atrophy. While some are cognitively normal before seizure onset, ID eventually develops in all affected individuals and the majority have severe cognitive impairment. Affected individuals have prominent comorbidities including ASD and motor symptoms such as hypo-

Box 3 *A female infant presented with epileptic spasms at age 10 months, associated with developmental regression. Prior to seizure onset, her development was mildly delayed. Prior to the genetic diagnosis, she was treated with oxcarbazepine, which led to exacerbation of seizures. At age 15 months, a heterozygous, de novo likely pathogenic variant in SCN2A was identified by WES. Treatment with ketogenic diet, vigabatrin, and ACTH improved cognition and development and temporarily resolved seizures, but epileptic spasms recurred after weaning ACTH. Additional antiseizure medications (levetiracetam, valproic acid) were not effective. At age six years, while treated with clobazam, clonazepam, and phenobarbital, she experienced up to three seizures per day. She had generalized hypotonia and did not sit independently or reach for objects. She turned her head toward sounds and made nonspecific vocalizations. Additional medical issues included intermittent choreoathetosis, autonomic dysfunction (periodic flushing with Raynaud-type phenomenon in hands and feet, constipation), mouthing, and leg-crossing stereotypes.*

tonia, choreiform, or dyskinetic movement disorders. A representative clinical description is illustrated in Box 3.

Later onset DEE associated with pathogenic *SCN2A* variants has a notable genotype–phenotype relationship [42]. Typically, *SCN2A* variants in this cohort are reported to have loss-of-function (LOF) effects due to missense, protein truncating, and splice site variants or missense variants with mixed GOF/LOF effects [15]. For example, the mixed function p.R853Q variant is the most common recurrent *SCN2A* variant [42]. Individuals carrying this variant present with a characteristic phenotype consisting of epileptic spasms, hypsarrhythmia on EEG, and choreiform movement disorder [42,43,44].

In *SCN2A*-related disorders associated with LOF variants, seizures are typic-ally treatment refractory and seizure freedom occurs in only 34 percent of cases [5]. Seizures are typically unresponsive to sodium channel blockers and can worsen after the introduction of this class of antiseizure medication. Persons with later onset DEE respond better to other drug classes including benzodi-azepines, levetiracetam, sodium valproate, and ACTH, compared with early onset DEE [15]. Specific later onset DEE phenotypes associated with patho-genic *SCN2A* variants are described next.

Infantile Epileptic Spasms Syndrome (IESS)

A prominent phenotype associated with *SCN2A*-related later infantile onset DEE is IESS [5,42]. Typical interictal EEG features include hypsarrhythmia or multifocal or focal epileptiform discharges, which may occur soon after the onset of epileptic spasms [13]. Age of onset is typically between 3 and 24 months. Developmental delay is observed after onset of epileptic spasms, but may be absent early in the course. Abnormal neurological examination findings may be present including abnormalities of posture, tone, or movement. The family, pregnancy, and birth histories are usually normal. Cognition varies from normal to severely delayed before seizure onset; however, moderate to pro-found developmental impairment becomes evident with time [13,15]. Long-term prognosis is unfavorable and many subsequently evolve to LGS [5]. *SCN2A*-related IESS is difficult to treat and does not respond to standard antiseizure medications, steroids, or ketogenic diet [5,34].

The main differential diagnoses for late onset IESS are other genetic etiolo-gies including pathogenic variants in *ARX*, *IQSEC2*, *TSC1*, *TSC2*, and others [13]. For early onset IESS, *CDKL5* and *STXBP1* should be considered [13]. In addition, a range of chromosomal abnormalities and copy number variants has been associated with IESS [45,46,47].

SCN2A-Related Disorders without Epilepsy

Individuals with pathogenic variants in *SCN2A* may present with NDD without epileptic seizures. The proportion of *SCN2A*-related disorders without epilepsy is unclear because of an ascertainment bias arising from preferential genetic testing of children presenting with seizures as compared with children having non-syndromic ID. Perhaps the best estimate of the incidence comes from the DDD study [48]. Inclusion criteria for the DDD study were broad, including children with severe undiagnosed NDD and/or congenital anomalies, abnormal growth parameters, dysmorphic features, and unusual behavioral phenotypes [7]. Richardson et al. reported the phenotypes of 22 persons including 12 presenting with neonatal or early infantile (≤3 months) onset seizures, four with ID/ASD and later onset seizures (seizure onset between two and nine years), and six with ID/ASD that had no history of epilepsy or epileptic seizures [48]. Thus, it could be estimated that approximately 20–30 percent of persons with NDD associated with *SCN2A* variants have no history of epileptic seizures.

In the large series of 201 individuals with *SCN2A*-associated disorders, 16 percent did not have epileptic seizures, although this sample may have ascertainment bias [5]. In the Richardson et al. study, all participants with either later onset seizures or no history of seizures had de novo variants and most (6 of 10) were protein truncating [48]. In contrast, all variants associated with the early onset seizure phenotypes (≤3 months) were missense. Among the six study participants without epilepsy, the degree of ID varied from mild to profound; half were formally diagnosed with ASD and no one had ataxia. Normal or nonspecific neuroimaging findings, including cerebral atrophy and hypoplasia of the corpus callosum, were reported for this subset. EEG findings were not reported by Richardson et al. [48], but a case report described the EEG in the setting of later onset developmental delay without epilepsy associated with a de novo missense *SCN2A* variant [49]. Findings in this case were bilateral discharges of high amplitude sharp waves and slow waves in the parietal–temporal–occipital regions that increased during sleep and were associated with right frontal-central short sequences of 5–4 Hz spike and wave complexes.

Episodic Ataxia

Episodic ataxia is observed in a subset of individuals with pathogenic *SCN2A* variants [50,51,52,53]. Most have epileptic seizures beginning during the first three months of life, and all have missense variants in the gene, suggesting that episodic ataxia may be a GOF disorder related to the early onset epilepsy phenotype. Onset of ataxia ranges from 10 months to 14 years. Episodes are highly variable, ranging from brief daily events to infrequent long-lasting episodes. Acetazolamide was effective in only a minority of reported cases [53]. In a systematic review of genetic epilepsies associated with paroxysmal ataxia, potential triggers for paroxysms of ataxia in *SCN2A*-related disorders were cited including minor head injuries, sleep deprivation, alcohol ingestion, photic stimulation, sudden noise, vibration of the body, and menstruation [54]. The majority (80 percent) with *SCN2A*-related episodic ataxia have good cognitive outcomes. A clinical vignette describing this syndrome is presented in Box 4.

In addition to episodic ataxia, other paroxysmal movement disorders have been anecdotally associated with *SCN2A* variants, including paroxysmal dyskinesia and choreoathetosis occurring in the context of both early and later onset

Box 4 *A female patient with an uncomplicated prenatal and perinatal history developed focal clonic seizures beginning on the fifth day of life. These were controlled with intravenous phenytoin and did not recur. Starting at age 10 months, she developed episodes of marked truncal ataxia, lasting 12–24 hours and occurring twice per month. Introduction of carbamazepine (titrated up to 10 mg/kg twice daily) and acetazolamide (titrated up to 2 mg/kg three times daily) did not change the frequency or severity of the episodes. At age two years she had a mild global developmental delay and muscular hypotonia. She was found to have a de novo pathogenic missense variant in* SCN2A.

epilepsy [50,55,56]. Severe choreoathetosis has been reported in persons heterozygous for the recurrent *SCN2A* variant p.R853Q [12,43,44]. Familial and sporadic hemiplegic migraine has also been associated with pathogenic *SCN2A* missense variants either with no history of epilepsy or with SeLFNIE [57]. Alternating hemiplegia of childhood has also been associated with pathogenic *SCN2A* variants in cases without mutations in the main gene (*ATP1A3*) [58].

There is no strong evidence supporting specific therapeutic approaches for patients with non-epileptic movement disorders associated with *SCN2A* variants. The majority of functionally tested variants associated with episodic ataxia exhibit GOF properties in either in silico or in vitro models. This is consistent with many cases being observed in the context of prior neonatal onset epileptic seizures. There are very few case reports of effective treatment of ataxia with sodium channel blocking medications. Treatment with acetazolamide has often been reported to be effective at reducing frequency and severity of ataxia episodes in approximately half of patients. Acetazolamide has been reported as effective in cases associated with both GOF and LOF variants in *SCN2A* [53].

Genotype–Phenotype Correlations

General genotype–phenotype correlations are established for *SCN2A*-related disorders. Individuals with self-limited epilepsy are heterozygous for mostly inherited missense variants [12]. More severe epilepsy phenotypes are mainly associated with de novo variants that confer greater electrophysiological dysfunction [12,59]. There are no clear correlations between the location of the variant on the protein and phenotypic severity. Amino acid substitutions between physicochemically similar amino acids are less likely to cause severe disease and are more frequently observed in self-limited epilepsies [12,60]. Functional analyses of some variants associated with self-limited epilepsy and episodic ataxia phenotypes have demonstrated GOF effects [51,53,61].

Individuals with early onset DEE mainly have missense variants (77 percent) but can also carry truncating variants (23 percent) [5,12,62]. The missense variants tend to cause GOF effects; however, the functional properties are complex and do not strictly separate as GOF or LOF based on age of epilepsy onset [63]. Truncating and nonsense (premature termination codon) variants present exclusively in individuals with seizure onset beyond the first year of life or without epilepsy, and those with truncating variants are reported to have seizures in 50 percent of cases [5,12]. The majority of individuals with truncating variants have features of ASD or developmental delay, compared to only 20 percent of those with missense variants. Individuals with ID/ASD and later onset epilepsy or absence of epilepsy mainly have truncating variants (75 percent) that are LOF [5,12,62].

Recurrent *SCN2A* variants occur throughout the phenotypic spectrum (see Table 1), but individual variants may not always associate with the same phenotype, even within families [5,64]. A computational analysis of clinical features of 413 individuals with pathogenic *SCN2A* variants demonstrated that only 8 of 62 individual recurrent variants were associated with similar phenotypes [42].

To date, the most frequently reported recurrent variants are p.R853Q (located in domain 2), p.A263V (in domain 1), and p.R1882Q (C-terminus) (Table 1). Of note, other amino acid substitutions have also been reported at the 1882 position, including p.R1882G/L/P, although these are not recurrent variants [5,51,65]. The p.R853Q variant is associated with later onset DEE characterized by IESS, severe ID, intractable seizures, and choreoathetosis [5,12,43], and less commonly with ASD [42,66]. Individuals heterozygous for p.R1882Q, which causes a strong GOF, had seizure onset on day of life one and at least one died of SUDEP [5,29]. Phenotype is more variable for other amino acid substitutions at this position. For example, p.R1882G is associated with self-limited epilepsy with later-evolving episodic ataxia [50,51,53]. The p.A263V variant is associated with early infantile DEE [5,67]. Two recurrent variants (p.E1211K, p.L1342P) are consistently associated with later onset DEE [66]. The LOF variant p.R937C is most often reported with a phenotype of developmental delay, ID, and/or ASD without seizures [66,68].

Table 1 Recurrent missense *SCN2A* variants (reported in four or more affected individuals)*

Variant	Number	Clinical phenotype	Location	Functional assessment / prediction
p.R853Q	18	EE [34,43,204] [5,44,205,206,207] NE [208]	Domain 2, S4 segment	Mixed/LOF [44,63,165,209] in silico prediction: LOF [121]
p.A263V	14	EI-DEE [5,37,51,53,210,211,212] SLE [50,52,53,67]	Domain 1, S5 segment	GOF [50] in silico prediction: GOF [121]
p.R1882Q	10	EI-DEE [5,29,44,212,213] LO-DEE [44]	C-terminus	GOF [5,44] [63,214] in silico prediction: GOF [121]
p.E999K	8	EI-DEE [5,34,213,215,216] LO-DEE [212]	Domain 2–3 linker	GOF [63,91,217] in silico prediction: neutral [121]
p.L1342P	5	LO-DEE [5,55,218,219]	Domain 3, S5 segment	Mixed [62] in silico prediction: GOF [121]
p.R1319Q	5	SLE [11] EI-DEE [5]	Domain 3, S4 segment	Mixed/LOF [63,220]
p.L1650P	4	LO-DEE [221] NE [221]	Domain 4, S4–5 linker	in silico prediction: GOF [121]
p.M1545V	4	EI-DEE [5,156,222,223]	Domain 4, S1 segment	in silico prediction: GOF [121]
p.R1629H	4	EI-DEE [5,206,212] SLE [206]	Domain 4, S4 segment	in silico prediction: GOF [121]
p.V261M	4	SLE [5,50] EI-DEE [206] LO-DEE [224]	Domain 1, S5 segment	GOF [50] in silico prediction: GOF [121]

* data adapted from Crawford et al. [42]

Abbreviations: ASD = autism spectrum disorder, EI-DEE = early infantile developmental and epileptic encephalopathy, GOF = gain of function, LO-DEE = later onset developmental and epileptic encephalopathy, LOF = loss of function, NE = non-epilepsy phenotype, SLE = self-limited epilepsy

Interpretation of *SCN2A* Variants

Interpretation of single nucleotide or copy number variants in *SCN2A* should be done in collaboration with a neurologist or geneticist with expertise in genetic variant interpretation. Features to be considered include: (1) frequency in population databases such as gnomAD,[1] (2) inheritance pattern, (3) similarity to previously described variants and/or if there are nearby pathogenic variants, (4) in silico predictions, and (5) consistency with described phenotypes. The SCN Portal,[2] ClinVar,[3] UniProt,[4] and publications provide valuable resources to determine if a variant is previously described and what clinical phenotypes are reported to determine where it is located relative to functional domains of the protein (see Figure 5B) and whether there is information on functional impact. Diagnostic laboratories will classify the variant as pathogenic, likely pathogenic, or a variant of uncertain significance based on standard guidelines [69,70,71]. Functional impact of novel variants cannot be definitively determined with bioinformatics tools.

The Biology of *SCN2A*

SCN2A encodes the voltage-gated sodium (Na_V) channel formally named $Na_V1.2$. The primary amino acid sequence of this protein was originally deduced from rat brain by complementary DNA (cDNA) cloning. Because it was the second sequenced brain Na_V channel sequenced, it was designated as rat brain type II. Functional studies of rat $Na_V1.2$ in *Xenopus* oocytes revealed a tetrodotoxin-sensitive, rapidly activating and inactivating inward current that resembled native neuron sodium currents [72,73]. The primary amino acid sequence of human Na_V 1.2 was determined in 1992 and its functional and pharmacological properties were similar to the rat channel [74]. The human *SCN2A* gene resides on the long arm of chromosome 2 (2q24.3) and consists of 27 exons spanning more than 150 kilobases.

Unlike voltage-gated potassium channels, which require assembly of tetramers (4 subunits) to function, Na_V channels are single polypeptides that form a pseudotetrameric arrangement of four similar domains (designated as I–IV or D1–D4) [75]. Each of the four domains consists of six transmembrane spanning segments (S1–S6), with the fourth transmembrane segment (S4) in each domain acting as the primary voltage sensor. Segments S5 and S6, along with the intervening pore (P)-loop of each domain, interact to form a conductive pathway selective for Na^+ ions (Figure 5). Sodium ion selectivity is conferred by aspartic acid (D), glutamic acid (E), lysine (K), and alanine (A) residues individually contributed by the four domains

---

[1] https://gnomad.broadinstitute.org   [2] https://scn-portal.broadinstitute.org
[3] www.ncbi.nlm.nih.gov/clinvar   [4] www.uniprot.org

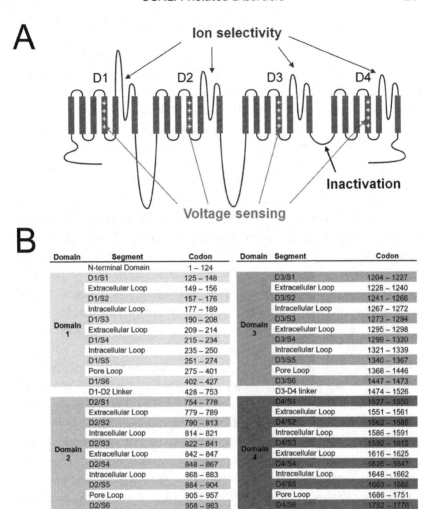

Figure 5 Transmembrane topology of a Na$_V$ channel. (A) Simplified structure of a Na$_V$ channel highlighting major functional domains. (B) Location by codon number of individual transmembrane segments and domains in Na$_V$1.2.

[76,77]. The III–IV cytoplasmic linker region, along with the C-terminal domain, are involved in channel inactivation [78,79,80]. During the three decades after sequencing the first brain Na$_V$ channels, many research groups worked to elucidate the structural, biophysical, and pharmacological properties of Na$_V$1.2 in great detail and investigated the underlying contribution of this channel to neuronal physiology in health and disease [81,82,83]. The protein structure of Na$_V$1.2 at atomic scale was determined using cryogenic electron microscopy [84].

Na$_V$1.2 Biophysical Properties

Na$_V$ channels mediate the initiation and propagation of APs [85]. Neuronal Na$_V$ channels, including Na$_V$1.2, have elaborate gating mechanisms that support rapid channel activation, inactivation, and recovery from inactivation, all of which are essential to sustain high-frequency AP firing. The sequence of events occurring during a neuronal AP is well understood (Box 5). The biophysical properties of Na$_V$1.2 that enable the AP include voltage-dependent and time-dependent (kinetic) properties. Voltage-dependence refers to the voltage range

---

Box 5 *Synaptic signals summing to produce a localized area of membrane depolarization (excitatory postsynaptic potential) of sufficient magnitude (threshold) elicits a sudden biphasic change in the membrane potential: first depolarization, then repolarization. The initial "upstroke" of the AP (depolarization phase) is caused by the opening of Na$_V$ channels. These channels are normally closed at the resting membrane potential but open (activate) upon a sufficiently strong local membrane depolarization. Activation of Na$_V$ channels is voltage-dependent owing to intrinsic voltage-sensors that are part of the protein. Opening of Na$_V$ channels allows Na$^+$ to rush into the cell due to a favorable electrochemical gradient (high extracellular Na$^+$ concentration and negative cell interior). The rush of Na$^+$ into the cell causes the membrane potential to further depolarize toward the Na$^+$ equilibrium potential (E$_{Na}$), which is approximately + 60 mV in mammalian neurons. Almost immediately (1–2 msec) after opening, Na$_V$ channels undergo a conformational change that closes the ion conducting pore by a process called inactivation. Sodium channels remain inactive until the membrane is repolarized. This phenomenon is a major reason for the refractory period – a short time window following an AP during which a second AP cannot be stimulated at all (absolute refractory period) or can only be elicited using a stronger second stimulus (relative refractory period).*

(in millivolts) over which channels activate and inactivate, while kinetic properties describe the time scales (in milliseconds) during which these events occur.

Activation of Na$_V$ channels results in a transient, rapidly inactivating current, but in some situations a small amount of non-inactivating (persistent) current remains (Figure 6). Persistent sodium current is physiologically involved in neuronal pacemaking of CA1 pyramidal neurons driven by muscarinic stimulation, as well as amplification of synaptic signals from both excitatory and

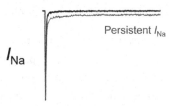

I_{Na}

Persistent I_{Na}

Figure 6 Representative voltage-clamp recording of wild-type (upper trace) and pathogenic variant Na_V channel with enhanced persistent sodium current (arrow).

inhibitory inputs [86,87,88]. Pathophysiologically, as will be discussed below, mutations that lead to abnormally large levels of persistent current can be associated with epilepsy.

$Na_V 1.2$ During Neurodevelopment

$Na_V 1.2$ undergoes developmentally regulated RNA splicing, resulting in two major channel isoforms with slightly different functional properties. This splicing event leads to the incorporation of an alternate exon 5 that encodes a portion of the domain I voltage sensor (S3 and S4 segments) [89,90]. The resulting neonatal and adult splice isoforms differ by a single amino acid residue at position 209 (asparagine in neonatal $Na_V 1.2$; aspartic acid in adult $Na_V 1.2$) and in some biophysical properties [91]. Analysis of gene expression data from rodents and primates demonstrated that during early prenatal and immediate postnatal brain development, $Na_V 1.2$ mRNA transcripts predominantly contain exon 5N (neonatal $Na_V 1.2$) [92,93]. Progressively through the first months of postnatal development, exon 5 splice-switching leads to predominant expression of transcripts containing exon 5A (adult $Na_V 1.2$). Neonatal $Na_V 1.2$ exhibits a depolarized voltage-dependence of activation, a hyperpolarized voltage-dependence of inactivation, and slower recovery from inactivation compared to the adult isoform. Given that immature neurons have a depolarized resting membrane potential compared with mature neurons, this combination of biophysical features would suggest that neonatal $Na_V 1.2$ may act to limit neuronal excitability during development [91,94]. To corroborate this, a mouse model engineered to express only adult $Na_V 1.2$ throughout development showed greater neuronal excitability and increased seizure susceptibility compared to wild-type (WT) littermates [95]. Thus, variants in $Na_V 1.2$ which show predominant GOF phenotypes may be particularly damaging during this critical period. Indeed, some variants exhibit exacerbated phenotypes in the neonatal isoform compared to that of the adult isoform [91].

Modulation and Regulation of Na$_V$1.2

Na$_V$1.2 activity is modulated by a number of factors, including protein–protein interactions, posttranslational modifications (e.g., phosphorylation, palmitoylation), and changes in intracellular Ca^{2+} concentration. Like other Na$_V$ channels, Na$_V$1.2 interacts with members of a family of nonconducting accessory β subunits that appear to modulate channel properties and promote forward trafficking to the plasma membrane [96,97,98]. Heterologous co-expression of the β1 and β2 subunits with Na$_V$1.2 results in larger peak current amplitude, shifts in the voltage-dependence of inactivation, and faster channel activation and inactivation. In addition to β subunits, Na$_V$1.2 also interacts with fibroblast growth homologous factors, which bind to the channel C-terminal domain. Members of this family of proteins have a range of effects on channel function. Co-expression with FGF13-1a (also known as FHF2a) results in larger current amplitude and enhanced frequency-dependent channel rundown, whereas FGF13-1b (also known as FHF2b) causes the channel to be more resistant to frequency-dependent rundown [99]. Additionally, FGF14-1b (also known as FHF4b) attenuates Na$_V$1.2 current amplitude [100].

Intracellular Ca^{2+} regulates Na$_V$1.2 by activating Ca^{2+}/calmodulin-dependent kinase II (CaMKII), which phosphorylates the channel. In the presence of activated CaMKII, the voltage-dependence of inactivation is significantly depolarized, and persistent current mediated by Na$_V$1.2 is larger, suggesting that CaMKII-mediated phosphorylation enhances channel function [101]. While calmodulin was shown to interact with the C-terminus of the channel, the functional consequences of this interaction are not well established [101,102].

Na$_V$1.2 also interacts with members of the ankyrin family, cytoskeletal proteins that promote cellular localization. In neocortical pyramidal neurons, ankyrin-G scaffolds Na$_V$1.2 to the axon initial segment (AIS) and nodes of Ranvier, whereas ankyrin-B scaffolds Na$_V$1.2 in dendrites [103,104].

Na$_V$1.2 Function in Cells and Circuits

Na$_V$1.2 channels are expressed throughout the central nervous system from the most ancient brainstem regions to the more recently evolved neocortex (Figure 7). There is an emerging understanding of Na$_V$1.2 function throughout development and how dysfunction of this important channel affects neuronal excitability and integrative properties of cells and circuits. Four Na$_V$ channel subtypes are expressed in the central nervous system (Na$_V$1.1, Na$_V$1.2, Na$_V$1.3, Na$_V$1.6), which are encoded by four distinct genes (*SCN1A*, *SCN2A*, *SCN3A*, *SCN8A*, respectively). While Na$_V$1.6 is present on the plasma membranes of

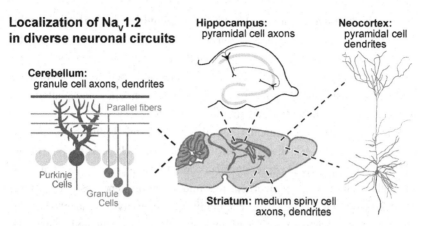

Localization of Na$_v$1.2 in diverse neuronal circuits

Cerebellum: granule cell axons, dendrites

Parallel fibers

Purkinje Cells

Granule Cells

Hippocampus: pyramidal cell axons

Neocortex: pyramidal cell dendrites

Striatum: medium spiny cell axons, dendrites

Figure 7 Localization of Na$_V$1.2 in diverse neuronal circuits. In mature circuits from mouse and rat models, Na$_V$1.2 expression within axons or dendrites largely corresponds to the presence of myelin. In cerebellum (left), Na$_V$1.2 is expressed in unmyelinated granule cell axons. In hippocampus (top), Na$_V$1.2 is expressed in unmyelinated axons of pyramidal cells. In neocortex (right), Na$_V$ 1.2 is expressed in somatodendritic compartments of pyramidal cells whose axons myelinated. In striatum (bottom), current data suggests that Na$_V$1.2 is expressed in all neuronal compartments.

a majority of neuronal classes, Na$_V$1.1 and Na$_V$1.2 appear to function in largely nonoverlapping groups [105,106,107,108,109,110]. Furthermore, Na$_V$1.2 expression within neurons varies by neuron type and at different time points during development. In mature neurons, Na$_V$1.2 localization is correlated with axonal myelination, with unmyelinated axons containing Na$_V$1.2 and myelinated axons excluding Na$_V$1.2 [111]. In the latter population, emerging evidence indicates that Na$_V$1.2 is present in dendrites [112,113]. As such, Na$_V$1.2 function can vary markedly across the brain, affecting either input or output structures of neurons.

Na$_V$1.2 function, and its relationship to other ion channel classes, has been studied most extensively in neocortical structures. *SCN2A* is transcriptionally expressed in a range of cell classes, including excitatory and inhibitory neurons [114]; however, this expression translates into Na$_V$1.2 predominantly in excitatory pyramidal neurons [109]. Within pyramidal neurons, the distribution of Na$_V$1.2 channels on the membrane changes during development. Early on, when neurons are still differentiating and elaborating neurites, Na$_V$1.2 appears to be the sole Na$_V$ channel expressed in pyramidal neurons [95]. This period spans the first year of life in humans and the first week of life in mice, a model system commonly used to study this channel. During this time period, Na$_V$1.2 is found at highest density at the AIS, the site of AP initiation [115]. Because AP initiation is supported by $Na_V1.2$ during this developmental period, genetic variants can affect overall neuronal excitability, resulting in hyper- or hypoexcitability in developing neocortical networks. Indeed, hyperexcitability in these circuits is considered etiological to early infantile epileptic encephalopathy, which occurs within the first few months of life [5,12,41].

After this early developmental period, Na_V channels redistribute. $Na_V1.6$ expression increases and displaces $Na_V1.2$ in the distal AIS and at axonal nodes of Ranvier [116]. $Na_V1.2$ expression also continues to increase [103], but these channels accumulate in neocortical pyramidal neuron dendrites [112]. Here, $Na_V1.2$ is critical for dendritic excitability and activity-dependent synaptic maturation and plasticity. Under normal conditions, APs initiated in the AIS propagate both forward to sites of neurotransmitter release and backward into the dendrite. The latter "backpropagation" is partly a passive process, limited by the electrical properties of dendritic cables, and partly supported by Na_V channels. As discussed below, heterozygous loss of *Scn2a*, which is associated with ID/ASD, impairs this backpropagation process, with downstream effects on synaptic maturation and plasticity.

In contrast to neocortical pyramidal neurons, $Na_V1.2$ is distributed differently in unmyelinated axons where, instead of being excluded, $Na_V1.2$ is enriched [111]. This distribution pattern is best understood in striatal medium spiny neurons [117], hippocampal pyramidal neurons [118,119], midbrain dopaminergic neurons [110], and cerebellar granule cells [120], but likely extends to other neuron classes with unmyelinated axons. Interestingly, AP threshold does not appear affected by heterozygous loss of $Na_V1.2$ in either hippocampal pyramidal neurons or cerebellar granule cells [120], indicating that another Na_V channel, presumably $Na_V1.6$, supports AP initiation in these cells. Instead, $Na_V1.2$ supports AP propagation, ensuring faithful transmission of those APs from the AIS to sites of neurotransmitter release.

Dysfunction of $Na_V1.2$

Detailed analysis of $Na_V1.2$ biophysical properties provides critical insight into how *SCN2A* variants can result in NDD. This work is typically done in heterologous expression systems, including human embryonic kidney cells (HEK293) that express few to no sodium channels of their own. Channel biophysical properties can then be studied using patch clamp recording. Thus, researchers have been able to quantify numerous biophysical features and assign binary classifications such as GOF or LOF to individual parameters. Data from such experiments in combination with other information such as

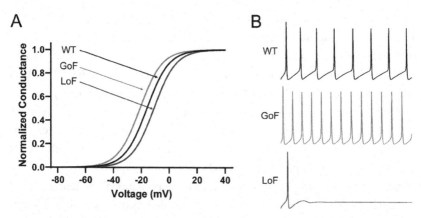

Figure 8 Effect of altered $Na_V1.2$ activation voltage-dependence on neuronal excitability. (A) Activation curves illustrating WT channels and variants with either GOF or LOF. (B) Simulated APs from a layer five cortical pyramidal neuron corresponding to the three conditions. Simulations performed with NEURON as described by Thompson et al. [91].

evolutionary conservation are also useful for training and validating computational (in silico) methods to predict the general functional effects of *SCN2A* variants [60,121,122].

One illustration of the GOF versus LOF concept is the effect of changes in voltage-dependence of activation on neuronal excitability (Figure 8). As stated earlier, $Na_V1.2$ channels are activated by membrane depolarization. Any mutation that hyperpolarizes the voltage-dependence of activation would increase the number of APs fired by a given stimulus, resulting in neuronal hyperactivity. By contrast, a depolarizing shift in activation voltage-dependence would result in fewer APs and neuronal hypoactivity. One can predict that mutations that enable channel opening at weaker stimulus intensities, cause channels to remain open longer, or recover faster from inactivation will potentiate neuronal excitability. Conversely, mutations that require stronger stimuli or result in channels that prefer nonconducting states would lower neuronal excitability.

Characterization of a limited number of variants has suggested that Na_V 1.2 variants with strong GOF properties result in early onset epileptic encephalopathies, while LOF variants are associated with later onset epilepsies, ASD, or non-syndromic ID [5,66,68,91]. Some variants fall neatly into these two divergent categories. For example, T236S was identified in a child diagnosed with early infantile epileptic encephalopathy (Ohtahara syndrome) and showed a large hyperpolarizing shift in the voltage-dependence of activation, consistent with GOF [91]. Other biophysical abnormalities interpreted to be GOF include enhanced persistent sodium current and slower onset of inactivation, which result in greater magnitudes of Na^+ influx over time. By contrast, the ASD-associated variant R937H is an example of a nonconducting $Na_V 1.2$ variant [68]. However, many $Na_V 1.2$ variants associated with neurodevelopmental diseases do not exhibit simple binary effects on channel function. Instead, many mutations exhibit a constellation of GOF and LOF properties, making the net effect on neuronal output difficult to predict [63].

Additional experimental strategies such as computational modeling of APs and dynamic AP clamp can help predict the net effects of $Na_V 1.2$ dysfunction on neuronal excitability (Figure 9). In silico prediction of neuron excitability by simulating neuronal APs computationally has informed the impact of certain variants on neuronal excitability [68,91], and efforts to scale this method for higher throughput are underway [123]. Dynamic AP clamp interfaces voltage-clamp recording of a heterologously expressed $Na_V 1.2$ variant with a computational model of a neuron or of an isolated neuronal domain such as the AIS. This approach has been used to predict effects of $Na_V 1.2$ variants on the propensity of an AIS model to generate APs [44,66]. Beyond these approaches, expressing $Na_V 1.2$ variants in native neurons may be the ultimate solution for determining pathogenic effects. The technology of using induced pluripotent stem cells (iPSC) to generate genetically defined human neurons is emerging as a new approach to assess the impact of $Na_V 1.2$ variants on neuronal firing behavior [124,125]. To date, only a limited number of studies have demonstrated effects of either GOF or LOF variants [126,127,128]. Importantly, cultured iPSC-derived neurons exhibit features comparable to an embryonic state, which may be a limitation for modeling disorders with postnatal onset. Transgenic and knockin mouse models are covered in the next section.

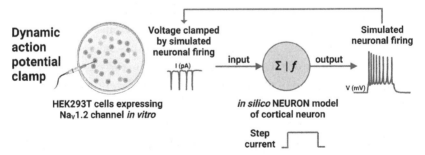

Figure 9 Illustration of dynamic AP clamp.

SCN2A in Epilepsy

Initial reports of an association of *SCN2A* with human epilepsy came from family studies of benign familial neonatal-infantile seizures, which was renamed SeLFNIE in recognition that seizures are not always benign [13]. In 2002, *SCN2A* variants were found to segregate with epilepsy in two independent multi-generational pedigrees [10]. The clinical spectrum expanded to include *SCN2A*-associated DEE with the first reported associations in 2009 [129,130]. SeLFNIE is a transient disorder with seizure onset in infancy that resolves after two years of age and responds well to sodium channel blockers. Inherited SeLFNIE variants are less deleterious than de novo variants associated with DEE. *SCN2A*-related DEE can be separated by age of seizure onset. Early seizure onset before three months of age is associated with GOF variants that respond to sodium channel blockers, while later seizure onset after three months of age is associated with partial or complete LOF variants that are exacerbated by sodium channel blockers. More details on the genotype–phenotype relationships in *SCN2A*-related disorders were covered the Clinical Spectrum and Genotype–Phenotype Correlations section.

The first mouse model of *SCN2A*-related epilepsy preceded the association with human epilepsy and provided supportive evidence for those early reports. $Scn2a^{Q54}$ mice express a transgene in neurons with a GOF missense mutation that results in elevated persistent sodium current in vivo and a severe epilepsy phenotype [131]. Phenotype severity in $Scn2a^{Q54}$ mice is dependent on background strain, supporting a contribution of genetic modifiers even in the case of a highly penetrant driver mutation [132]. $Scn2a^{Q54}$ mice have been a useful system for identifying genetic modifiers that may contribute to variable presentation of epilepsy associated with *SCN2A* variants [101,133,134,135]. With the advent of genome editing technology, it has become easier to develop knockin models carrying human pathogenic variants in the corresponding position in the mouse gene. New mouse models of *SCN2A*-related disorders have been reported, including those with recurrent variants for early onset and later onset DEE [136,137]. $Scn2a^{R1882Q}$ mice, carrying the most recurrent early onset DEE variant, exhibit a severe phenotype, with seizure onset in the neonatal period and premature lethality by postnatal day 30. Pyramidal neurons from $Scn2a^{R1882Q}$ mice exhibit higher evoked AP firing frequency, higher input resistance and lower rheobase, consistent with a GOF phenotype [136]. In contrast, $Scn2a^{R853Q}$ mice, carrying the most recurrent later onset DEE variant, had no spontaneous seizures or EEG abnormalities and were less prone to seizures induced by chemoconvulsants [137]. Primary cortical neurons from $Scn2a^{R853Q}$ mice showed lower firing frequency and less network bursting compared to WT neurons, consistent with a LOF phenotype [137].

Pathogenic variants exhibiting mixtures of LOF and GOF properties make it challenging to translate in vitro biophysical defects into a predicted effect on neuronal excitability. One such mixed function *SCN2A* variant is K1422E, which exhibits altered ion selectivity allowing partial Ca^{2+} permeation and lower overall conductance [76,77,138]. A child carrying this variant presented with developmental delay, epileptic spasms with onset at 13 months of age, and features of ASD [139]. Consistent with the mixed effects on channel function, $Scn2a^{K1422E}$ mice exhibit a combination of GOF and LOF phenotypes, including rare spontaneous seizures, background EEG abnormalities, and altered thresholds for induced seizures, as well altered neurobehavior that overlaps features of *Scn2a* haploinsufficient mice [138]. Recordings from layer 5b pyramidal neurons showed impaired AP initiation and larger intracellular Ca^{2+} transients at the AIS during the rising phase of the AP, consistent with a complex effect of the p.K1422E variant on neurons. The complex effects of mixed-effect variants suggests that therapeutic responses may be challenging to predict for these special cases. Additionally, genome background and biological sex have been shown to influence phenotype severity in $Scn2a^{K1422E}$ mice [138,140,141], adding to the complexity.

SCN2A in Autism Spectrum Disorder and Intellectual Disability

SCN2A variants were first associated with ASD in 2012 in a landmark genetic analysis of exomes of 928 individuals, including 200 phenotypically discordant sibling pairs [142]. In this cohort, *SCN2A* was the only gene found to have disruptive de novo variants in two separate ASD cases, which was deemed extremely unlikely due to chance. In the decade following, the association of *SCN2A* with ASD strengthened, and the gene is now recognized as the leading genetic risk factor for ASD among all genes identified by exome sequencing [143,144]. This large-scale effort was conducted by the International Autism Sequencing Consortium. One of the lead investigators was Matthew State, PhD, Professor and Chair of Psychiatry and Behavioral Sciences, University of California, San Francisco, who was interviewed for this Element by Kevin Bender, PhD (Video 2).

Despite this strong ASD association, unraveling the contributions of *SCN2A* to ASD has not been straightforward. Of the 72 genes currently associated with ASD, *SCN2A* was initially considered an outlier, because most genes encode proteins that localized to or regulate synapses or are genes encoding chromatin modifiers in neuronal nuclei [144]. By contrast, *SCN2A* encodes a Na_V channel involved in AP initiation and propagation in neuronal axons, which was considered distinct from synapses and gene regulatory processes in the nucleus. It

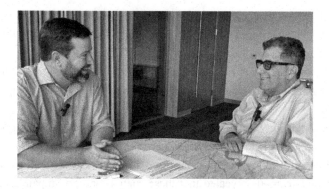

Video 2 Two-part discussion with Matthew State, MD, PhD (Professor and Chair, Department of Psychiatry and Behavioral Sciences, University of California, San Francisco) moderated by Kevin Bender, PhD (Associate Professor of Neurology, University of California, San Francisco) on discovery of *SCN2A* as a risk gene for ASD, the neurobiology of this gene, and prospects for future treatments. Transcripts of these videos are available in the Appendix. The video files are available at www.cambridge.org/scn2a

was with the discovery that $Na_V1.2$ localizes to neocortical pyramidal cell dendrites that some level of convergence was first understood. In dendrites, $Na_V1.2$ interacts functionally with synaptic genes, regulating dendritic excitability and synaptic plasticity. Heterozygous loss of $Na_V1.2$ in neocortical neurons results in cell-autonomous impairments in dendritic excitability. This dendritic excitability is instructive for activity-dependent refinement of excitatory circuits. In heterozygous *Scn2a* knockout (*Scn2a$^{+/-}$*) mice, excitatory synapses are less mature, with an excess of silent synapses, lower AMPA: NMDA receptor ratio, and greater proportion of NR2B-containing NMDA receptors more commonly found in developing synapses. Furthermore, impairments in Na_V-supported propagation of APs into the dendritic compartment were associated with a failure to induce synaptic plasticity [103,112]. Evidence has emerged that ankyrin-B, encoded by the ASD-risk gene *ANK2*, contributes to scaffolding $Na_V1.2$ channels to dendritic membranes. Heterozygous loss of ankyrin-B in mice phenocopies the synaptic dysfunction discovered in *Scn2a$^{+/-}$* mice, and this implicates dendritic dysfunction as a convergent mechanism in ASD.

Impairments in synaptic plasticity also extend to other brain regions in *Scn2a* haploinsufficiency. In hippocampus and cerebellum, excitatory synapses onto principal neurons (pyramidal cells and Purkinje cells, respectively) can be strengthened in response to bursts of input at high frequency. In both brain regions, the axons that convey these bursts are unmyelinated and use $Na_V1.2$ to propagate APs from the AIS to synaptic boutons. In $Scn2a^{+/-}$ mice, this transmission may be less reliable, simply because there are fewer Na_V channels available to initiate APs [145]. As a result, synaptic plasticity that depends on burst transmission is either blunted or eliminated in both brain regions [119,120].

Synaptic plasticity deficits may be linked to behavior. Although $Scn2a^{+/-}$ mice perform reasonably well in many behavioral assays [112], they may have difficulties performing more complex spatial memory tasks. Unit recordings from the hippocampus revealed that these spatial memory impairments were correlated with alterations in "replay," which is a coordinated, sequential activation of a series of hippocampal pyramidal neurons that appears associated with the animal recalling its movement through space [146]. Moreover, recent work examining cerebellar circuitry has revealed that $Scn2a^{+/-}$ mice and children heterozygous for *SCN2A* LOF variants exhibit hypersensitivity of the vestibulo-ocular reflex (VOR) [120]. The VOR is a conserved behavior that reflexively moves the eyes in the opposite direction of the head to help stabilize a visual scene on the retina. In mice, the combination of heightened VOR sensitivity and an inability to modulate VOR amplitude is linked specifically to heterozygous loss of *Scn2a* in cerebellar granule cells, which are neurons that provide excitatory input to Purkinje cells, and was found to impair synaptic plasticity between granule cells and Purkinje cells. This form of plasticity is common throughout the cerebellum [147]. As such, deficits in VOR behavior may serve as a bellwether of broader dysfunction in cerebellar plasticity, which could affect a range of behaviors, including motor coordination and social interaction [148].

Mouse genetics allows for study of not only *Scn2a* haploinsufficiency, mimicking the condition resulting from heterozygous LOF variants, but also genetic conditions not observed in humans (Figure 10). While constitutive knockout of *Scn2a* is lethal [149], 75 percent loss of *Scn2a* throughout the brain, or conditional knockout of *Scn2a* in select neuron classes, is tolerated [113,150]. These conditions have helped reveal phenotypes not easily observed in heterozygous $Scn2a^{+/-}$ mice that may nevertheless inform on the human condition. To generate 75 percent loss of *Scn2a*, a gene knockdown approach termed gene trap was used to block most transcription from both *Scn2a* alleles in mice [151]. These mice display a range of behavioral deficits not observed in heterozygous $Scn2a^{+/-}$ mice, including markedly elevated anxiety-related behavior, impaired nesting behavior, and fractured sleep associated with altered activity in the suprachiasmatic nucleus [151,152]. Moreover, ex vivo recordings of principal neurons in striatum and neocortex revealed an unexpected intrinsic

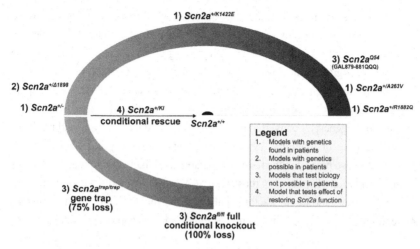

Figure 10 Range of Na$_V$1.2 dysfunction in reported mouse models of *SCN2A*-related disorders. Mouse models with genotypes and phenotypes associated with *SCN2A*-related disorders span and expand on the range of genotypes observed in the human population. GOF missense variants include those observed in children (black) and those that result in epilepsy in mice due to knockin of amino acids that would be unlikely to occur in humans (Q54). Mixed function variants, with features of both GOF and LOF, have been generated for the K1422E variant, which converts Na$_V$1.2 from a Na$^+$ ion selective channel to a nonselective cation channel. LOF variants include variants that truncate the Na$_V$1.2 protein. Beyond these cases that can occur in children, mouse genetics has allowed for other approaches, including ~75 percent to 100 percent reduction of *Scn2a* expression, either throughout the brain or in select cells, as well as rescue alleles where full *Scn2a* expression can be restored in neurons using Cre recombinase.

hyperexcitability in AP generation, which was due to lower potassium channel function that normally dampens excitability. Hyperexcitability was also observed when *Scn2a* expression was completely knocked out using a viral approach in adolescent mice (postnatal days 28–44). In this case, hyperexcitability was due not to a change in potassium channel expression but rather to a disrupted interaction between the loss of dendritic Na$_V$1.2 and dendritic potassium channels, where a loss of Na$_V$1.2-mediated depolarization led to a loss of potassium channel-mediated repolarization. Because neurons did not hyperpolarize to the same voltages between APs, it was then easier to generate subsequent APs [113]. Such effects appear consistent in vivo, as conditional knockout in the same population of pyramidal cells, and only those pyramidal cells, is sufficient to promote seizures [153].

Overall, these changes in excitability, observed when model systems are pushed beyond heterozygosity, may shed light on why some children with *SCN2A* protein truncating variants develop epilepsy. They suggest that *Scn2a*$^{+/-}$ mice, on the C57BL/6 background, are near a threshold for excess excitability that can be observed if the system is pushed. Of note, different strains of inbred mice display different propensity for seizures and can be either protective or more susceptible to seizure electrogenesis if converted into an epilepsy model (e.g., by providing a pro-convulsant drug or making a genetic manipulation to a key ion channel). This variability is also present in the human population and likely contributes to variability in presentation of epilepsy in those with *SCN2A* LOF variants. Moving forward, a deeper understanding of factors that push or pull systems from a seizure susceptibility cliff will be critical, in both mouse models and other model species.

Treatment of *SCN2A*-Related Disorders

Treatment of *SCN2A*-related disorders is primarily aimed at seizure control along with supportive therapies for symptoms related to ASD and developmental delay. When possible, treatment should to be tailored to an individual's pathogenic variant. Certain strategies such as the use of sodium channel blocking antiseizure medications may be more effective in persons with GOF variants and less effective in cases with LOF variants. While symptomatic treatments will continue to be important, disease-modifying therapeutic strategies targeting the underlying pathophysiology are emerging. This section will initially focus on the symptomatic treatment of epilepsy followed by a discussion of emerging disease-modifying therapies for which preclinical proof-of-concept exists for *SCN2A*-related disorders.

Antiseizure Therapy for *SCN2A*-Related Disorders

Epilepsy due to GOF variants typically presents as neonatal or early infantile onset seizures. Clinical evidence supports the notion that sodium channel blockers are more often effective in this setting, but are less effective or ineffective if epilepsy begins after three months of age [5]. The difference in epilepsy age of onset between groups with GOF versus LOF variants is a general trend but is not absolute, and some variants are difficult to categorize because they exhibit features of both GOF and LOF [63].

The efficacy of specific sodium channel blockers in the setting *SCN2A* GOF variant is heterogeneous. In a limited number of case series, phenytoin and carbamazepine had the best response rates [5,154,155]. High dose phenytoin may be required for efficacy [154,156], but this is accompanied by greater risk of adverse effects and requires close monitoring of plasma free drug concentration. Awareness of potential drug–drug interactions and pharmaco-genomic factors is also important [157]. Genetic variants in CYP2C9 affecting phenytoin metabolism may predispose to toxicity [158]. While use of sodium channel blockers can produce significant seizure reduction in individuals with GOF variants, anecdotal evidence suggests developmental delays may persist [156,159].

Individuals with *SCN2A* LOF variants may also have seizures, which tend to begin later in infancy or in early childhood and do not generally respond to sodium channel blockers [5]. There is little evidence supporting specific antiseizure therapies for affected individuals with *SCN2A* LOF or mixed function variants. Treatment for *SCN2A*-related NDD is primarily supportive, with applied behavioral analysis along with physical, occupational, and speech therapies. Recognition of cortical visual impairment allows accommodations to be integrated into an individual's care plan in a way that maximizes successful visual interaction with their environment.

Emerging Disease-Modifying Therapies for GOF *SCN2A* Variants

While no disease-modifying therapy is currently available for *SCN2A*-related disorders, many potential avenues are being investigated (Table 2), with some

Table 2 Potential disease-modifying strategies for *SCN2A*-related disorders

Type of therapy	*SCN2A* GOF	*SCN2A* LOF
Small molecule drugs	persistent current blocker*	sodium channel activator[#]
Antisense oligonucleotides	gapmer/RNAseH*	poison exon (TANGO)[#]
Transcriptional modulation	CRISPR interference RNA interference	CRISPR activation*
Gene delivery	N/A	activating transcription factor[#] SCN2A transgene
Nonsense suppression	N/A	tRNA suppressor (targeting premature stop codon)
Gene editing	base editing, prime editing	base editing, prime editing

* existing preclinical proof-of-concept for *SCN2A*;
\# preclinical proof-of-concept for another sodium channel gene;
N/A, not applicable

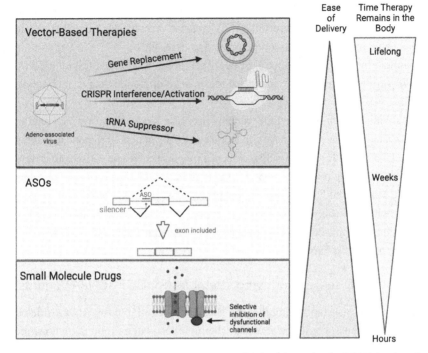

Figure 11 Overview of potential disease-modifying therapies in *SCN2A*-related disorders. The left side of the figure illustrates general approaches. The triangle on the right side illustrates the ease of delivery (most difficult delivery is the top). The inverted triangle on the right side illustrates the time therapy remains in the body. Created with BioRender.com.

moving into clinical trials. The remainder of this section will focus on emerging therapeutic approaches that may have efficacy for these conditions (Figure 11). These advances are made possible by collaborations between academic laboratories and the pharmaceutical industry, as illustrated by an interview with Dr. Steven Petrou, Professor of Translational Neuroscience, University of Melbourne, and Chief Scientific Officer of Praxis Precision Medicines (Video 3).

Small Molecule Drugs

Conventional drug therapy, which modulates the activity of mutant sodium channels, is the mainstay of treatment for *SCN2A* GOF variants. However, sodium channel blocking antiseizure medications such as phenytoin do not correct the underlying functional defect and also affect normal sodium channels. New small molecule drugs in development are attempting to target

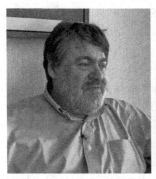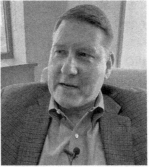

Video 3 Interview of Steven Petrou, PhD (Chief Scientific Officer, Praxis Precision Medicines) conducted by Alfred L. George, Jr., MD (Professor and Chair of Pharmacology, Northwestern University) explaining his transition from academic research to leading a new pharmaceutical company developing treatments for *SCN2A*-related disorders. A transcript of this video is available in the Appendix. The video file is available at www.cambridge.org/scn2a

channel dysfunction more precisely with the goal of being more effective with less toxicity.

One strategy targets a specific functional anomaly, enhanced persistent sodium current, exhibited by many *SCN2A* GOF variants. Persistent sodium current arises when channel inactivation is not complete, leading to a small level of inward current that can affect neuronal excitability. This functional anomaly occurs in many sodium channelopathies in addition to *SCN2A*-related disorders. The first animal model (Q54 mouse) to test the hypothesis that enhanced *SCN2A* persistent current can cause epilepsy was reported years before the first human mutations were discovered [131]. Later investigations using this mouse model demonstrated the antiseizure efficacy of an approved antianginal drug, ranolazine [160], which selectively suppresses persistent current carried by cardiac sodium channels [161]. This study was motivated by in vitro evidence that ranolazine blocked persistent sodium current carried by mutant $Na_V1.1$ channels (encoded by *SCN1A*) [162,163]. Acute exposure of Q54 mice to ranolazine was effective at reducing seizure frequency, but poor brain penetration indicated that this drug would not be effective clinically [161]. However, a novel nonselective sodium channel blocker (GS-458967 or GS967; later named PRAX-330) was described as a potent and preferential inhibitor of persistent sodium current [164]. GS967 exhibits near complete seizure suppression in Q54 mice and prevented seizures following maximum electroshock [160]. GS967 was shown to suppress persistent current carried by recombinant human $Na_V1.2$ [165] and to prevent seizures in a mouse model of DEE caused by an *SCN8A* GOF variant [166,167].

Despite success in mouse models, GS967 had undesirable pharmacokinetic properties (e.g., excessive plasma and brain half-life) [164] and exhibits potent use-dependent block of peak sodium current [168]. However, the observed efficacy of preferential persistent sodium current block in mouse models of epilepsy motivated development of newer agents, including PRAX-562 [169] and NBI-921352 [170], although neither was selective for $Na_V1.2$. PRAX-562 is orally active and exhibits greater preference for blocking persistent current carried by mutant or neurotoxin (ATX-II)-modified $Na_V1.6$ channels than conventional sodium channel blocking antiseizure drugs (e.g., phenytoin, carbamazepine, lamotrigine) [169]. This compound has similar effects on other human sodium channels, including $Na_V1.2$. By contrast, NBI-921352 is selective for blocking $Na_V1.6$ channels and doesn't specifically target persistent current [170]. In mice subjected to maximum electroshock, PRAX-562 exhibits dose-dependent anticonvulsant effects with less neurotoxicity than carbamazepine and lamotrigine [169]. Following demonstration of tolerability in healthy volunteers [171], PRAX-562 received orphan drug and rare pediatric disease designations by the FDA and entered Phase 2 clinical trials for *SCN2A*- and *SCN8A*-related DEE (NCT05818553, ClinicalTrials.gov).

While more targeted drugs show promise for controlling epilepsy, there remains the question of whether this type of therapy will be disease-modifying because sodium channel blockade has not been shown to rescue the neurodevelopmental phenotype. In theory, this could be related to the degree of selectivity for the mutant sodium channel and whether the small molecule corrects the specific pathophysiology of a particular pathogenic variant. It is conceivable that more precise sodium channel inhibition initiated earlier in the disease course may potentially improve seizure control and developmental outcomes.

Antisense Oligonucleotide (ASO)

Among the first disease-modifying therapies approved for NDD was an ASO (nusinersen) for spinal muscular atrophy [172,173]. ASOs are short stretches of synthetic nucleic acids typically comprised of deoxyribonucleic acid (DNA) or chemically modified ribonucleic acid (RNA) nucleotides. These nucleic acid drugs bind to a complementary sequence (antisense) within mRNA or pre-mRNA and act either by steric interference with enzymatic processing (e.g., splicing, translation) or by engaging ribonuclease H (RNaseH) to cleave hybrid RNA:DNA duplexes. Chemically modified RNA nucleotides (e.g., ribose-O-2-methoxyethyl or 2'-MOE) coupled with sulfur-containing (e.g., phosphorothioate) backbone linkages are employed to shield the molecule from degrading enzymes [174]. ASOs used to target mRNA or pre-mRNA for RNaseH cleavage typically use a 'gapmer' design consisting of a DNA core (needed to form nuclease-susceptible RNA:DNA duplexes with the target) flanked by short chemically modified RNA sequences (Figure 12). Splice-modifying ASOs can be composed of DNA or modified RNA only. These two mechanisms of action make ASOs versatile in their application (Figure 13), leading to several clinical trials for a variety of neurogenetic conditions [175,176,177,178].

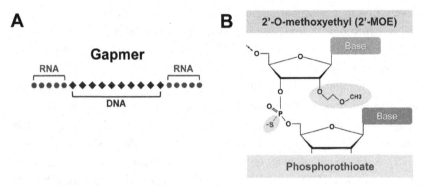

Figure 12 Design features and chemistry of a gapmer ASO. (A) Gapmer design with a 10 nucleotide DNA core and flanking five nucleotide modified RNA sequences. (B) Chemical structure of a 2'-MOE RNA base with phosphorothioate linkage.

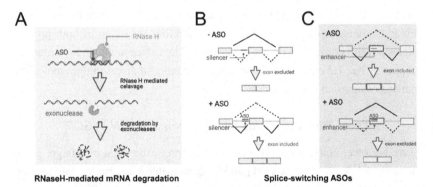

Figure 13 Strategies for gene regulation by ASOs. (A) RNase H–mediated mRNA degradation. (B) Splice-switching ASOs that promote exon inclusion by masking silencer regions. (C) Splice-switching ASOs that promote exon skipping by masking splicing enhancer regions. Adapted from Carvill et al. [176] and reproduced with permission from Springer Nature. Created with BioRender.com.

Preclinical evidence suggests that ASOs have potential therapeutic benefits for *SCN2A*-related disorders associated with GOF variants. Li et al. demonstrated that immediate postnatal delivery of a gapmer ASO targeting *SCN2A* by the intracerebroventricular route lowered spontaneous seizure frequency and prolonged survival in mice heterozygous for a GOF missense variant (equivalent to human R1882Q) [136]. Administration of the ASO two weeks after birth also conferred a survival benefit, as did a second dose given approximately four weeks after birth in mice that received a first dose on day one of life. The ASO used in this study did not affect protein levels of other neuronal sodium channels, and treated mice showed no overt neurological toxicity. In 2023, a human *SCN2A*-selective ASO (PRAX-222, elsunersen) entered early stage clinical trials (NCT05737784, ClinicalTrials.gov).

While encouraging, these results need to be taken with tempered expectations as there are important considerations with ASO treatment in this context. A potential concern is over-reduction of $Na_V1.2$ protein levels, which may induce a LOF phenotype, a concept referred to as the goldilocks principle [179]. ASOs do not allow for quick or easy dose titration given their long half-lives (more than 100 days in brain), and this creates challenges for achieving a specific range of mRNA and protein reduction. Uptake in brain is not uniform, with superficial structures and spinal cord having higher uptake than deep structures [180]. Another consideration is whether a simple reduction in $Na_V1.2$ protein will result in the appropriate level of functioning protein. The ASO will down-regulate both *SCN2A* mRNA alleles. It is important to recognize that while we refer to variants that result in increased currents as "gain-of-function," this is dysfunctional sodium current, and therefore reduction of both protein alleles doesn't correct the defect specifically. The extent to which lowering the amount of $Na_V1.2$ channels will produce a meaningful disease improvement in humans remains an open question.

Other Potential Therapeutic Strategies for SCN2A GOF

There are other emerging approaches for lowering expression of a target gene, including RNA interference [181] and programmable transcription interference using clustered regularly interspaced short palindromic repeat (CRISPR) interference [182] that could have value for *SCN2A* GOF variants [183]. These approaches could work in a similar way as ASOs to diminish $Na_V1.2$ channel production. In addition to suppressing expression, base editing [184] and prime editing [185] are promising technologies for correcting pathogenic variants, which have been successful for other genes and may work in mammalian brain [186].

Emerging Disease-Modifying Therapies for LOF *SCN2A* Variants

CRISPR-Cas9 Activation (CRISPRa)

As mentioned earlier, CRISPR technology can enable targeted transcriptional regulation of genes. In the original embodiment, a CRISPR-associated nuclease (e.g., Cas9) cleaves genomic DNA at a position targeted by a single guide RNA (sgRNA), creating double-stranded breaks that are repaired by either nonhomologous end-joining or homology-dependent repair. An enzymatically inactive Cas9 ("dead" Cas9, dCas9) or a chimeric dCas9 fused to a transcriptional activator can similarly be positioned at a precise location in the genome, but this will not cut DNA. Rather, placing the chimeric dCas9 near the transcription start site will activate transcription for that gene. This strategy, called CRISPR activation (CRISPRa) [182], has been demonstrated to boost *SCN2A* expression in heterozygous knockout mice and human stem cell-derived neurons [187]. In that study, CRISPRa components were delivered in vivo using recombinant adeno-associated virus (AAV) intravenously or by stereotaxic injection directly into mouse brain. CRISPRa restored normal neuronal and dendritic excitability in heterozygous mice and did not induce seizures in WT mice. The latter observation suggests there are regulatory mechanisms to prevent *SCN2A* overexpression, which could convert a LOF disorder into a GOF disorder. Similar success has been demonstrated for *SCN1A* LOF in a mouse model of Dravet syndrome [188].

An alternative approach for transcriptional activation of brain sodium channel genes involves use of engineered transcription factors. This approach has been used successfully for boosting neuronal expression of *SCN1A* and improving survival of Dravet syndrome mice [189]. Preparations for an early phase clinical trial with the molecule used in this study (ETX101) commenced in 2022 (NCT05419492, ClinicalTrials.gov).

Other Potential Therapeutic Strategies for SCN2A LOF

Preclinical proof-of-concept exists for additional approaches for rescuing LOF variants in other sodium channel genes. Targeted augmentation of nuclear gene output (TANGO) is a strategy for suppressing unproductive mRNA splicing events arising from inclusion of "poison exons," which evoke nonsense-mediated decay. Unproductive splicing events involve several genes associated with NDD [190], including *SCN1A*, which encodes the $Na_V1.1$ sodium channel and is the major gene responsible for Dravet syndrome. A splice-switching ASO (STK-001) prevents inclusion of a poison exon in *SCN1A* transcripts, boosts translation of functional $Na_V1.1$ protein, and improves survival in a Dravet syndrome mouse model [191,192]. Clinical trials are underway to test efficacy and safety of STK-001 in

Dravet syndrome (NCT04442295, NCT04740476, ClinicalTrials.gov). Whether a similar strategy will work for *SCN2A* LOF variants is unknown.

Hypothetically, *SCN2A*-related disorders caused by LOF variants could be approached by delivering an exogenous copy of the recombinant gene or its coding region to brain using a viral vector. While conceptually appealing, this approach is not feasible with the currently available vectors that are most advanced in clinical trials (e.g., AAV), because the large size of the *SCN2A* coding region exceeds the capacity of these vectors. Newer vectors may overcome this size restriction as demonstrated for *SCN1A* [193,194,195].

For *SCN2A* LOF variants that create premature termination codons (PTC, nonsense), a novel approach (nonsense suppression) utilizing modified transfer RNA (tRNA) may have value. This approach seeks to trick ribosomes into incorporating the correct amino acid at the location of the PTC by using anticodon engineered tRNA molecules [196,197]. Intrinsic features of the translational machinery appear to protect native stop codons from the modified tRNA. Viral delivery of a suppressor tRNA was used successfully in vivo in mice to partially correct an engineered PTC mutation in the gene encoding α-1-iduronidase, which causes the lysosomal storage disease mucopolysaccharidosis type I in humans [198]. Nonsense suppression has garnered considerable commercial interest [199] and there is interest in applying this strategy for *SCN1A* and *SCN2A* [195,200], but major challenges must be overcome [197].

Considerations for Disease-Modifying Clinical Trial Design

Bringing a disease-modifying therapy to the clinic requires not only evidence of efficacy but also a need to consider aspects of clinical trial readiness. These include precise clinical trial design (duration, most appropriate control group), accurate patient selection (age, variant type), and outcome measures that can demonstrate meaningful changes over time. Clinical trials for conventional small molecule drugs with a primary seizure endpoint are based on established designs, such as randomized, placebo-controlled trials, but these are less feasible and appropriate for disease-modifying therapies [201]. Furthermore, for *SCN2A*-related disorders disease-modifying therapies may target specific subsets of affected individuals, which further subdivides an already rare disease and may compromise study power.

Variations from traditional clinical trial designs are required to achieve well-powered studies. One nontraditional trial design, stepped-wedge design (also known as a randomized start design) [201], has specific advantages such as allowing comparison both within groups and between groups, thereby increasing the power of the study with a relatively small number of trial participants. Using this approach, all groups eventually receive treatment, which is ethically superior to trials with a placebo group. The effect of treatment duration can also be investigated because each group is introduced to the treatment at different time points. So-called "n of 1" trial designs, including individual crossover studies, may also have value in rare diseases [202]. Depending on the chosen outcome measures, study duration may need to be adjusted to account for developmental outcomes that require longer study times. Careful consideration of these features is needed for clinical trial designs in *SCN2A*-related disorders to ensure collection of the rich and diverse data necessary for successful assessment of a novel therapy.

Another challenge to clinical trial design in *SCN2A*-related disorders is the heterogeneous functional effects of variants. As described previously, specific strategies can be tailored to either GOF or LOF variants. While neonatal and early infantile-onset epilepsy is typically associated with GOF variants, this is not absolute. For the aforementioned clinical trial of an ASO for *SCN2A* GOF variants (PRAX-222), study participants must have seizure onset before three months of age (NCT05737784, ClinicalTrials.gov). However, this could potentially include some affected individuals with LOF variants unknown at the time of enrollment. For future disease-modifying therapies, especially with approaches with permanent effects such as gene delivery and gene editing, functional testing of variants prior to treatment may need to be considered [122]. Furthermore, individuals in this and other *SCN2A*-related clinical trials are enrolled beginning at age two years, which is well beyond disease onset and raises the possibility that response to therapy could be affected by prior seizure burden or pharmacological treatments.

Selection of appropriate clinical trial outcome measures is challenging for *SCN2A*-related disorders using existing methods. This is illustrated by a recent *SCN2A* clinical trial readiness study in which mean standardized domain scores on the Vineland Adaptive Behavior Scales were three standard deviations below the normative average [203]. The Vineland has challenges assessing small changes at low scores, and therefore raw scores or growth scale values may be more effective in eliciting meaningful change without a floor effect. Seizure reduction, even greater than a 50 percent reduction, as the main outcome measure may not encapsulate the full array of disease-modifying effects families and clinicians are hoping to achieve with these therapies, which often involve more risk than traditional seizure medications. With invasive and potentially permanent types of treatment (Table 2), the benefit of such therapies needs to outweigh those risks. The hope is that the benefit from a disease-modifying therapy would entail more than reducing seizure frequency. Given that seizure control in *SCN2A*-related disorders does not necessarily rescue the developmental phenotype, it will be especially important to target other outcome measures, including developmental achievement, sleep, quality of life, and behavior, among others, to ensure that the full spectrum of disease-modifying effects is being assessed.

Abbreviations

AAV	adeno-associated virus
AIS	axon initial segment
AP	action potential
ASD	autism spectrum disorder
ASO	antisense oligonucleotide
Cas	CRISPR-associated nuclease
CRISPR	clustered regularly interspaced short palindromic repeat
CRISPRa	CRISPR activation
DDD	Deciphering Developmental Disorders study
DEE	developmental and epileptic encephalopathy
EEG	electroencephalography
EIMFS	epilepsy of infancy with migrating focal seizures
ESES	electrical status epilepticus during slow-wave sleep
FDA	Food and Drug Administration
GOF	gain of function
HRQoL	health-related quality of life
ID	intellectual disability
iPSC	induced pluripotent stem cells
IESS	infantile epileptic spasms syndrome
LGS	Lennox-Gastaut syndrome
LOF	loss of function
MAE	myoclonic atonic epilepsy
NDD	neurodevelopmental disorders
PTC	premature termination codons
SeLFNIE	self-limited familial neonatal-infantile epilepsy
sgRNA	single guide RNA
SUDEP	sudden unexpected death in epilepsy
TANGO	targeted augmentation of nuclear gene output
tRNA	transfer RNA
VOR	vestibulo-ocular reflex
WES	whole exome sequencing

Appendix

Transcript of Video 1: Interviews of parents of children with SCN2A-related disorders

Q: How did you feel when you received the diagnosis of SCN2A-related disorder (SRD)?

Sandya Crasta, Missouri, USA: I felt shattered and heart breaking. The doctors did not know anything about this diagnosis. They were new to it, too, but luckily they do give us the information of the *SCN2A* Foundation, and that was helpful.

Liz Hendrickx, Belgium: My world just fell apart. I didn't know what to do, didn't know where to look because in Belgium no one – there just aren't that many cases, so I couldn't compare. And the doctors told me not to Google it [laughter], so that was pretty scary.

Ashley Taylor, Texas, USA: I felt a very mixture of emotions. For the first 23 months of my son's life, he was very neurotypical, met his milestones and stuff; and so, seizures hit around 23 months, and within two months of those seizures hitting – and they were coming constantly – we got that diagnosis. So I felt very overwhelmed, still processing the seizures, and now we have this other diagnosis that is causing these seizures. So it was a little bit of excitement knowing that there's something that they can possibly treat, but at the same time scary that they knew very little about it.

Amy Richards, Maryland, USA: I was actually thrilled. It was such a relief to finally figure out what was wrong. I knew from infancy that something had to have been wrong. I mean, I always equated it to a juggling act, that something would fall in our laps and, oh, she has GI reflux; oh, she's got a tic-ing behavior; oh, she's got apraxia of speech; oh, she has double hip dysplasia. And I kept saying, so then, what is it? There has to be something underlying. I just want a name for it.

Q: What do you feel is the hardest part about SRD?

Charlotte's mom, Minnesota: Charlotte was very severe and was born having over 400 seizures a day, and she was very prone to illness, so spent over half of her life in the hospital and a lot of time intubated. And she suddenly declined as her life went on, and she had more and more seizures. And towards the end of it, she was in status most of the time and her brain wasn't functioning any more. And I would say the hard part for me was that I am basically an ICU nurse, and so I knew too much, and watching her go through those things, in my heart I knew what the outcome was going to be.

Ashley Taylor, Texas, USA: Stripping everything away that I had envisioned for my child, that I had to re-evaluate, like, what his future might look like; and watching him suffer and not being able to do anything about that. And he still pushes through with a smile, and so it's pretty – but it's challenging to know that there's nothing I can do about it at this moment.

Q: Do you believe in a cure for SRDs?

Sandya Crasta, Missouri, USA: I do, do strongly believe in a cure, especially because of the FamiliesSCN2A Foundation, where, you know, all the – many of the board members and the parents coming together to find a cure and fight for this cause.

Liz Hendrickx, Belgium: That's the main reason why we're here, why we're not giving up, why we're going across the globe to find people who understand, who are willing to work with us. That's why I'm screaming it off the rooftops, telling everyone, this is what my child has. I even tell every cab driver, every Uber driver. I'm like, I'm here for this. This is my daughter, she has this. I'm telling everyone who wants to hear.

Amy Richards, Maryland, USA: I do, I think there's going to be one. And like I said, I'm not 100 percent it's going to be in her lifetime, but I think there's going to be enough in her lifetime that her life gets better. But I definitely think someday, yes, there can be a cure. To think that she's only 13, and in that short amount of time we've gone from me saying, there's something wrong with this infant, just give me a name; to, we know what it is; to now, three years later, what's happening? It blows your mind. It's mind boggling. So yes, the amount of research that's being done, this is – yeah, there's a cure, it's going to happen.

Q: How have you been impacted by FamilieSCN2A Foundation?

Ashley Taylor, Texas, USA: Huge support system, knowing that I'm not alone, and that there are others that understand my struggle, and it's a judgment-free zone. And in the same sense, it's a source of hope because I see what the Foundation is doing, and it gives me hope that people care and they are trying to do something about the *SCN2A* mutation.

Charlotte's mom, Minnesota: I believe that the Foundation, the *SCN2A* Foundation provides a community of support for our families that gives families hope. And I am really excited at the research that they have initiated to start to look more into this and to get doctors, you know, excited about researching this disease; and putting money towards finding a cure, or at least a better quality of life for our kids.

Sandya Crasta, Missouri, USA: I or my family has been impacted because we've got this, you know, we've got the support of the families that are impacted through this *SCN2A*. We ask questions and we get answers that we don't get from our doctors or, you know, so we get that mental as well as just the emotional support from each other. Even coming to the conferences and learning about, you know, what the research has done, or just meeting other families, has been possible through the funding that is available through the *SCN2A* Foundation, for which I am very grateful.

Learn more about the FamilieSCN2A Foundation at www.scn2a.org.

Transcript of Video 2 (part 1): Interview of Matthew State, MD, PhD, by Kevin Bender, PhD

Kevin Bender (KB): Hello, my name is Kevin Bender. I am a Professor in the Department of Neurology here at UCSF, and it is my honor and pleasure to be talking with Dr. Matt State, who is a human geneticist and child psychiatrist and also the Department Chair of Psychiatry and Behavioral Sciences here at UCSF. And we are hoping to have a nice chat about *SCN2A* and its role in autism spectrum disorder (ASD). Matt and Matt's group have been at the forefront of human genetics in trying to understand genetic underpinnings or genetic contributions to neurodevelopmental and neuropsychiatric disorders like autism spectrum disorder, and has made some very pivotal and, I would say, foundational discoveries on the contribution of rare de novo variants in genes like *SCN2A*, and has really opened up this field, which I think actually recently we called it the decade of gene discovery in ASD. And it's actually completely changed how we think about this disorder and how we can look at it and hope to develop therapeutics in the future. So, thank you, Matt, for having me today.

Matthew State (MS): It's an honor and a pleasure right back at you.

KB: Yeah. So, how did this start? How did you guys get started with this concept? Because I think it was a controversial idea to think about de novo variants, where there is a new change in genetics in a child that wasn't present in their parents, that is contributing to a disorder like ASD.

MS: I think, so – that's largely the case, I think. So, you know, we began working with a particular strategy, trying to find the kinds of mutations that you're talking about underlying common forms of psychiatric disorders. And I had a particular interest as a child psychiatrist in neurodevelopmental disorders, working with kids with autism and Tourette's syndrome, etc. So, you know, at that time, which was really at the turn of the millennium, the conventional wisdom was that psychiatric disorders were all uniformly genetically complex and that they were going to be a consequence of common variation in the genome, sort of hundreds to thousands of different spots in the genome contributing, each one, very small, individual effects. And for a variety of reasons, I came to the study of genetics with a kind of different perspective, that was really focused on using genetics as an entrée to understand neurobiology. So as opposed to trying to figure out sort of all of autism or understand the genetic architecture of neuropsychiatric disorders, all of which are very worthwhile and interesting things to do, I had a really kind of laser-like focus on what I used to say was, if I can just find one gene that I'm absolutely confident leads to autism – because we didn't have that in 2000, or at least not one that we were confident led to "idiopathic autism," so, autism without other features of severe neurodevelopmental problems. So honestly, the reason that, you know, I came to it that way because I have sort of a backwards educational path. I had completed all of my clinical training, was not a scientist, and decided to go back and do a PhD, and I did it specifically because I was seeing these kids on the units and lamenting every day the fact that we had no idea what was going on at the molecular level. So, sort of this sort of reductionist idea that, if I can just find one gene, that we can then begin to pull on that thread to go from genes to understanding, you know, cellular or molecular mechanisms in biology. So, all of this was aimed at this idea that we are, you know, sort of, if we can just find . . .

KB: Find that one gene.

MS: Yes, just the one gene. So then we got totally lucky, and it turned out that, in fact, much more of the disorder was underlaid by these kinds of mutations, but the things we were able to look for were, for a variety of reasons – we started looking at chromosomal breaks, and particularly looking for de novo chromosomal breaks in families in which it looked like a lightning strike genetically and we had a light microscope, that was kind of the only way to look across the genome to do this; but, you know, it's better to be lucky than to be good. I ended up at a place where we were developing tools to be able to screen the genome at much higher resolution looking for these mutations. And so by 2008 or 2009, we knew that there were changes in chromosomal structure that were contributing to idiopathic autism, that de novo rare mutations were doing that, again to a much higher rate; you know, it wasn't like the one in a million kids, it was more like 5 to 10 percent of kids. And then the ability to sequence the coding portion of the genome came through.

So, that was kind of the evolution of the strategy. And the critical milestone in about 2012 was, you know, we were all racing, a bunch of labs, and three hit the finish line exactly at the same time in a series of papers in *Nature* that showed that using this approach, that you could find rare de novo mutations that were damaging to the encoded protein, easily predict that because they were stop codons or, you know, clearly things that were damaging the protein; that they were carrying very significant risks, which is, you know, one piece of the many surprises that we found. And then, as it so happened, the first gene that we identified using this approach was *SCN2A*.

KB: Actually, if I remember correctly in that 2012 paper, that cohort was about how large, it was about 5,000?

MS: No, no, it was much smaller.

KB: Much smaller.

MS: Right. So, I mean that was . . .

KB: And even within that, you identified *SCN2A* twice.

MS: Yes.

KB: Which seems like astronomical odds. To be able to identify one gene – you hit one gene actually two times in a very small cohort.

MS: Yeah, so, that's exactly right. I love that that, like that was your reaction, because everyone else's reaction was, the cohort size was only about 200 . . .

KB: Oh, only 200.

MS: Yes. Well, you know, there were multiple groups, and each group had about 200 families that they were doing. So the issue is that, you know, the smaller the effect, the bigger the sample size you need. So the fact that we were able to find this among 200 represents how much of an impact mutation in *SCN2A* have in a kid, which is like – that was our ideal, right? We wanted to find something that had big, big biological effects.

KB: This was a case where you actually caught the same lightning bolt or two bits of the same lightning bolt in the same bottle . . .

MS: Yes.

KB: . . . in this cohort of 200 kids.

MS: Yes.

KB: Since then, it's now been 10 years, where the cohorts have gone larger and larger and larger, from 200 now I think to 60,000?

MS: Yes.

KB: Where has *SCN2A* fallen within this group? As the ability to actually look at this quantitatively has improved, where has *SCN2A* fallen?

MS: Yeah, it's at the very – I mean it, you know, it's turned out to be one of the most frequent among the group of genes that have rare de novo mutations, and that's how they're contributing to autism; and it's turned out to have very, very large individual effects, exactly what sort of this initial hit was suggesting. And in fact, so, there were three labs that published simultaneously; three genes came out of that: *CHDA*, a gene called *GRIN2B*, and *SCN2A*. All three of those – so, it just goes to show you that, you know, it's not completely random; we caught the lightning in the bottle because this is one of the more frequent with the largest effect size, so you can plausibly find it in 200 people. So, you know, again, it's always better to be lucky than good, it's good to be both, and in this case, you know, it was a harbinger of, you know, an overall strategy, but the gene ended up being in a whole variety of ways particularly valuable. Like, that combination of being relatively frequent and, for a rare mutation, and having such large effects; like that is absolutely the ideal . . .

KB: Never happens.

MS: Yeah, and you know, like I said, I came to this a kind of reformed clinician, right? With an idea that I was going to use genetics to ultimately try to get something, some knowledge that would be, that ultimately would translate into the clinic and impact. You know, again, when I started, it was like if I could know the biology in a way that would allow us to develop a treatment, even if it was for one family, two families, three families, that that would be enormous given how mysterious autism was 20 years ago and still is today. And so, you know, it's turned out in a whole variety of ways that *SCN2A* really presents, I think continues to present extraordinary opportunities.

So, once we found the gene, you know, we were incredibly excited. But then there were these whole series of kind of relatively quick-in-succession discoveries about *SCN2A* that, you know, that made it sort of this remarkable stroke of luck. So, at one point, I can't remember where, I called it the Rosetta stone, or potentially Rosetta stone for understanding autism.

KB: So, what do you mean by that?

MS: Yeah, yeah. So, the first is, is like, you know, it kind of would have been enough, just the fact that it was like one of the first genes, and you could think about the fact that having, you know – there were very few, in fact no psychiatric disorders at that time, apart from autism, where you could say, I have a rare mutation in coding portion of the gene and carrying very large effects that's causing a common neuropsychiatric or neurodevelopmental disorder. We didn't have that at the time. So, you know, like you would think, that could be enough to call it a Rosetta stone; but then it turned out, you know, that it actually really in terms of thinking about, could you elaborate biology from that finding? There are all these other characteristics that we found about the gene that really lead,

I think, to extraordinary opportunities to disentangle really complicated biology. So, one of them was that, in general, as we found these things – first I mentioned we found that rare changes in chromosomal structure could lead to autism; but at the same time what we found is that the same rare chromosomal abnormality not only led to autism but could lead to a whole variety of different neurodevelopmental outcomes. And, you know, that was an extraordinary, you know, observation, kind of defied our diagnostic nosology in psychiatry; but it also kind of presents some immediate challenges to think about, okay? I thought, well, if you have this rare gene, you're going to be able to pull on the thread; if the thread goes in 17 different directions simultaneously, you've got a problem, right?

KB: Yeah.

MS: So, and then with genes that we've identified, to some degree we found the same, actually to a large degree we found the same kind of underlying theme, which was that they were autism genes but they also were neurodevelopmental genes. But what was even kind of more complicating is that the kinds of mutations that we were finding didn't kind of give you immediate traction on seeing whether or not you could dissect, like, why does this one gene not only lead to autism but also lead in some cases to epilepsy, for instance?

KB: Yes, very, very commonly.

MS: Yes, very, very common, so about, particularly for kids – in general in autism, about 30 percent of kids will have epilepsy, but particularly for these rare, large-effect mutations you see a lot of overlap with epilepsy. So what was immediately – well, not immediately, but pretty soon after the discovery cooled – and actually this was Stephan Sanders, who was in the lab, he was a post-doc at the time and was the lead author on the gene discovery paper, was really interested in taking a look at the range of mutations that we were finding. And what was really unusual about *SNC2A* is that it started to look like there might be something really specific or much more specific than any other gene that we had, about this connection between the mutation, the kind of mutation in the gene and the outcome. So, there, again, like the notion that it could be a Rosetta stone, not only to begin to understand idiopathic autism but to really get traction on the biology of how does a rare mutation that causes a range of neurodevelopmental problems in some people end up being epilepsy, in others autism, in others the overlap of epilepsy of autism? Which turns out to be an incredibly interesting story.

Transcript of Video 2 (part 2): Interview of Matthew State, MD, PhD, by Kevin Bender, PhD

Kevin Bender (KB): I still remember the first time I met you was actually down at a retreat for our neuroscience program, and you got up and gave this wonderful talk. You had just moved with Stephan [Sanders] and Jeremy Willsey, all of you moved from Yale, take over as Chair of Psychiatry and Behavioral Sciences. And it was this watershed moment for me, sitting in the back of the room where you're displaying this huge map of genes associated with autism that you've just recently discovered. And there was this group that was modifying the transcription profile of neurons, and then there was this other group that was modifying synaptic transmission. And then you made this offhand comment; it was just like, oh yeah, and then we have this other gene, *SCN2A*, no idea what it does; it's down here in an axon and we don't know why it's there, but we can't ignore it. And I chase you down afterwards and you said, oh, hi, who are you? I said, I really want to work on this, and this was actually a moment where we got a chance to meet up, chat with Stephan, and it really started to dissect and to link the genetics to areas of biology.

And so, one of the first things we needed to do was actually characterize a lot of the variants that you had identified, and Stephan identified, within autism spectrum disorder; and they almost invariably led to loss of function, where the channel doesn't work as well as it should. And we had a really simple idea. It was, okay, it's a sodium channel, it's involved in generating action potentials; so therefore, these cells are not firing as well as they should, end of story. It was only when we got a mouse that recapitulates those phenotypes that, again, we were more lucky than good. We were completely surprised by what the biology was telling us, and that was – this is biology that we'd been doing since about 2016, 2017, where we're starting to unravel that it's not really the initiation of an action potential; it's actually the communication back to synapses, and those synapses that are really providing the inputs to neurons, especially in neocortex; and *SCN2A* is there to provide some communication, some crosstalk, some linking of activity and activity-dependent plasticity and all of these processes that are involved in learning – *SCN2A* is really supporting that mechanism. And so what we found invariably, both us, other labs throughout the US and abroad, we basically found that *SCN2A*, when you lose half of *SCN2A*, as happens in autism spectrum disorder, you have these very pronounced deficits of learning, and pronounced deficits in the forms of learning that we think might be closer to things that would manifest as ASD than other forms – so, things that are involved in generalization, really complex, abstract thought; things that are involved in social communication and understanding very subtle cues when you're having a conversation with someone. And it's really trying to understand what the biology that has been disrupted – it's been really remarkable that *SCN2A* has been able to teach us this.

One of the things that we found over and over again is this situation where, when you've lost half of your *SCN2A* expression, many neurons within the brain appear to stay in this pre-critical period holding point; and it's almost like they're waiting for the activity-dependent refinement, the activity-dependent plasticity to occur, but it just can't occur because you've lost *SCN2A*. And so that actually opens up an opportunity, I think, because what we've seen is that that holding period seems to be very, very extended in development. And it opens up the possibility that if we can restore *SCN2A*, in some way . . .

Matthew State (MS): Yes.

KB: . . . even late in development, we might be able to develop therapeutics that could reinvigorate plasticity mechanisms and allow for some sort of therapeutics.

MS: Yes.

KB: Because one of the problems – the thing that I struggle with as a neurophysiologist who now, who has been studying action potentials in a dark room for the last two decades, with no interaction with humans – I work with mice, I work with rats! – now meeting these families and meeting these lovely kids, these kids are only getting older . . .

MS: Yeah.

KB: . . . and we're not helping them yet.

MS: Yes.

KB: And so, understanding the windows of opportunity for treatment of disorders like this is something that's outrageously critical. And my question for you is, where – what should we do as biologists within the next five years or so, and where do you see the field of gene discovery and gene identification translating into therapeutic opportunities for the field?

MS: I think that there's a possibility that *SCN2A* is one of those perfect targets for a whole variety of reasons. And then this, you know, the notion about this overlap in phenotype, I think is actually going to be key to progress in the clinic now. And the reason is that – it's a long story that I won't belabor today, but the bottom line is that doing clinical studies of core deficits in autism is extremely difficult if not impossible right now in a way that's relevant for the FDA. That we don't know how to measure social behavior . . .

KB: Yes.

MS: ... in a way that is reliable enough in humans, and we can't do it in a timeframe – I'm not sure how well we can do it ever, but we definitely can't do it in a timeframe that might be relevant to measure in the clinic to say, oh, if we fix this gene we're fixing social development.

KB: Um-hmm.

MS: And therefore, what we can do is, we can study epilepsy.

KB: Yes, yes.

MS: And so the opportunity, because there is overlap, strong overlap between autism and epilepsy, I think in the next five years is going to be the path towards moving from basic biology to the clinic. There are a whole variety of things that are happening around interventions that are now plausible, including targeting individual genes either with, you know, gene replacement or in some cases antisense oligonucleotides. There are a variety of ways even potentially with repurposed small molecules if you can target epilepsy. It is now, you know, that is mature enough, work in that area is mature enough.

KB: Yeah, so that's the potential inroads to be able to ...

MS: Correct. I think I'm much more optimistic that we both in the next five years are going to begin to see evidence of the kind of work that we've both done ...

KB: Um-hmm.

MS: ... and be able to really start doing bench-to-bedside work; that there're going to be human trials that are going to give access to biology that we've never had before, that we're going to have animal models we're going to be able to really test whether or not our predictions based on animal, you know, being able to rescue in a model system, how that plays out, you know.

KB: Yeah.

MS: So, I think it's incredibly fertile ground.

Transcript of Video 3: Interview of Steven Petrou, PhD, by Alfred L. George, Jr., MD

Al George (AG): I'm conducting an interview today with Steve Petrou, the Professor of Translational Neurosciences at University of Melbourne, and also past Director of the Florey Institute for Neurosciences there. He is also, importantly, co-founder and now Chief Scientific Officer of Praxis Precision Medicines, which has devoted a tremendous amount of energy into developing new treatments for *SCN2A* disorders. Steve, thank you very much for doing this interview with us.

Steve Petrou (SP): Thanks for inviting me, Al, today; delighted to be here.

AG: The first thing I think people watching this video will be interested in knowing is, what first got you interested in studying *SCN2A*, and what were the driving questions at that time?

SP: Great question. I mean, my background really was in hard-core ion channel biophysics, all single-channel recordings, and when I set up my laboratory, I met Sam Berkovic and got very interested in mechanisms of disease mechanisms in genetic epilepsy. And the first area I got into was GABA, and then after studying GABA, and we made a mouse model, we were thinking very much about, well, what's the yin and yang of the brain, and the E and the I,[a] and obviously, you know, sodium channels and $Na_V1.2$, 1.6 were very important channels in determining inter-neuron and pyramidal cell function. So that said, there's a core biological interest in it. And then we started seeing information around the variants at that time responsible for a disorder called BFNIS [benign familial neonatal-infantile seizures], it's now called self-limiting epilepsy of infancy or neonatal/infancy. And then that was interesting from a basic biology perspective because I was always very, very interested in the work on the *drosophila* channels and how they used the phenotype to inform the function of the Shaker, Shab, Shal, Shaw family of channels. And this sort of gave me an opportunity to say, well, you know, human biology, genetics, has done the experiment to some extent, and so how do we understand dysfunction from that perspective in really well validated mutations? So we started studying the *SCN2A* at that point, and that was really before all the sporadic cases and the rare epilepsies started to be revealed, of course other than Dravet, which we knew about at the time. So that was my sort of starting point.

AG: So, can you think back to when you first started studying *SCN2A* variants in the benign familial neonatal/infantile seizure syndrome, which was brand new, there were so few variants; did you think this was going to last?

SP: No. I just thought we're going to just, we did a few GABAs, we've now done a sodium channel, there'll be, you know, a handful – there was only three or four different genes to choose from at the time. It wasn't a very big list.

---

[a] E and I refer to excitation and inhibition

I didn't think it was going to last. We really were thinking more about familial epilepsy, and then we also knew at the time that these, they were still very rare, these families. So the BFNIS families weren't a common form of familial epilepsy, you know, in the overall scheme of epilepsy. So thinking a lot about, how is this going to be impactful more broadly in the disease? And so, didn't think it was going to last, to be honest, and didn't think 20 years later, I'd still be doing it!

AG: What was the inspiration for then deciding to start a company? And take us back to the inspiration for starting Praxis, which I recall was not originally called Praxis; that's its newest name.[b]

SP: Right.

AG: Tell us that story, if you will.

SP: When I came back from my post-doc in the US into Australia and started my laboratory, I immediately got a part-time position as a VP of CNS Research at a small Australian startup called Bionomics. And that's where all the IP that Sam Berkovic and Grant Sutherland were generating around the familial epilepsies was residing; and we were thinking there at the time, well, how do we use that knowledge to deliver better therapeutics? And so, for me, that's where the whole concept – and that was in the early 2000s, you know, where the whole concept of around precision medicine. I think, you know, we were on, at the time, having knowledge of a mutation that was in one family in the world wasn't very useful. So, and efforts to try and see whether they could be broadened weren't that successful in common epilepsy. But it did teach me a lot about thinking how to turn science into impact. It wasn't really commercialization that interested me, it never really – you know, it's an important thing to do, but I've always been interested in seeing whether my research can be more impactful than just getting more h-factors and citations and papers. That was never enough of a driver for me personally. So, that was a big motivator. And that converted into consulting I did with other companies, ran a screening program for another US company for many years doing drug discovery.

AG: So, working with industry was not a foreign concept; it was natural, and it was a vehicle to maybe perhaps make more of a translational impact.

SP: It really was something that I'd always been doing, and I think, you know, later as the field matured, it became more and more apparent what you should do in that space.

[b.] Praxis was formerly named EpiPM Therapeutics when it was originally founded in 2015

AG: Steve, tell us about your interactions with *SCN2A* families and, in particular, the families that engaged with you to help move forward in translational activities in *SCN2A*?

SP: A great question, Al. It really was a convergence of several things: our continued interest in work on the biophysics of *SCN2A* mutations in sporadic childhood epilepsies; our beginning to make a mouse model of one of those mutations; and our interest in precision therapies. We sort of started, reached out to Ionis, thinking about how we want to apply ASOs to that arm, to the 2A gain-of-function cases; and at the same time, really, they reached out to me, the parents reached out to me, and we actually met at an AES meeting in the US when I visited and started to talk about what we were doing. They'd just got a fairly recent diagnosis and were very interested and were very, very motivated to try and do things. And so what they did do is really provide, they're now catalysts for really accelerating the delivery of precision medicine therapeutics. I was interested in proof-of-concept study with Ionis,[c] thinking, you know, how might we show that an ASO could be effective in an animal model as a potential for a future clinical program; but they said, let's think about what it would take to do the clinical program now.

AG: Based on all this trajectory, it was interesting to those of us in the field that you made the transition almost full time to industry now as Chief Scientific Officer of Praxis. And so, a couple things: What was the motivator for doing that? And what's your perspective on how different academic research and industry activities are?

SP: It became more and more apparent to me that my natural interest and desire is to really translate; and whilst I loved, and I still do, basic research, I still manage my laboratory, it really wasn't enough for me to just continue along that academic path. So I did want to see what it would take, and see whether I can actually influence the rate at which we can move these programs forward. So that was really what made me – and you know, with all the knowledge I've had around disease modeling, you know, the new genetics coming in, there was a lot of activity and thinking around precision medicine at the time as well, and I think at the White House had an initiative on precision medicine at the time as well. So, it was sort of a perfect storm to try and launch a company like that. And so that was really the catalyst for getting the company going; and then, you know, thinking about it for four or five years really did cement the idea that I want to go full time, you know, flip my work – now I'm more or less full time at

---

[c] Ionis Pharmaceuticals

Praxis, and I have a little small secondment to keep the laboratory going at Melbourne as well.

AG: Well, as we're drawing to the end of this interview, I want to just give you the chance to conclude by telling us what you're most excited about for the future of *SCN2A*?

SP: You know, I think we're starting to see the signs of it already, and that is a more nuanced understanding of how variants actually produce the clinical heterogeneity that we're seeing today. And it's obvious to me that it's never as simple as you first realize. The fact that we're seeing the same variant in a benign case versus a very serious case tells us that there's not only mechanistic complexity at the neuronal and the network and the whole-brain level, but there's always modifying effects as well. And I think what would be interesting to me is really understanding a very tight relationship between genotype and phenotype, understanding–developing a causal chain of understanding across the whole brain so we really maybe begin to understand where the pathologies that give rise to an early onset, a late onset, an autism, an autism with epilepsy – where does that pathology really emerge? And does it give us new opportunities for therapeutic intervention beyond the blocker for gain-of-function, up-regulator for loss of function; there might be new opportunities. And sort of related to that, I think, so once we develop that more nuanced understanding of the disease biology, I think there will be clear impacts beyond 2A epilepsy, and this will probably impact other brain disorders, depression and anxiety and a whole host of other things that will gain, you know, a lot of knowledge, and the lessons learned will be able to be applied to those other areas.

References

1. A. H. Poduri, A. L. George, Jr., E. L. Heinzen, D. Lowenstein, S. James, *How we got to where we're going*, A. H. Poduri, editor (Cambridge, UK: Cambridge University Press; 2021).

2. S. R. Cohen, I. Helbig, M. C. Kaufman, L. Schust Myers, L. Conway, K. L. Helbig, Caregiver assessment of quality of life in individuals with genetic developmental and epileptic encephalopathies, *Dev Med Child Neurol*, 64 (2022), 957–64. DOI: https://10.1111/dmcn.15187.

3. J. D. Symonds, A. McTague, Epilepsy and developmental disorders: Next generation sequencing in the clinic, *Eur J Paediatr Neurol*, 24 (2020), 15–23. DOI: https://10.1016/j.ejpn.2019.12.008.

4. J. D. Symonds, S. M. Zuberi, K. Stewart, et al., Incidence and phenotypes of childhood-onset genetic epilepsies: A prospective population-based national cohort, *Brain*, 142 (2019), 2303–18. DOI: https://10.1093/brain/awz195.

5. M. Wolff, K. M. Johannesen, U. B. S. Hedrich, S. Masnada, G. Rubboli, E. Gardella, et al., Genetic and phenotypic heterogeneity suggest thera-peutic implications in SCN2A-related disorders, *Brain*, 140 (2017), 1316–36. DOI: https://10.1093/brain/awx054.

6. T. W. Fitzgerald, S. S. Gerety, W. D. Jones, M. van Kogelenberg, D. A. King, J. McRae, et al., Large-scale discovery of novel genetic causes of developmental disorders, *Nature*, 519 (2015), 223–8. DOI: https://10.1038/nature14135.

7. J. F. McRae, S. Clayton, T. W. Fitzgerald, J. Kaplanis, E. Prigmore, D. Rajan, et al., Prevalence and architecture of de novo mutations in developmental disorders, *Nature*, 542 (2017), 433–8. DOI: https://10.1038/nature21062.

8. Q. Zeng, Y. Yang, J. Duan, X. Niu, Y. Chen, D. Wang, et al., SCN2A-related epilepsy: The phenotypic spectrum, treatment and prognosis, *Front Mol Neurosci*, 15 (2022), 809951. DOI: https://10.3389/fnmol.2022.809951.

9. M. B. Stosser, A. S. Lindy, E. Butler, K. Retterer, C. M. Piccirillo-Stosser, G. Richard, et al., High frequency of mosaic pathogenic variants in genes causing epilepsy-related neurodevelopmental disorders, *Genet Med*, 20 (2018), 403–10. DOI: https://10.1038/gim.2017.114.

10. S. E. Heron, K. M. Crossland, E. Andermann, H. A. Phillips, A. J. Hall, A. Bleasel, et al., Sodium-channel defects in benign familial neonatal-infantile

seizures, *Lancet*, 360 (2002), 851–2. DOI: https://10.1016/S0140-6736(02) 09968-3.

11. S. F. Berkovic, S. E. Heron, L. Giordano, C. Marini, R. Guerrini, R. E. Kaplan, et al., Benign familial neonatal-infantile seizures: Characterization of a new sodium channelopathy, *Ann Neurol*, 55 (2004), 550–7. DOI: https://10.1002/ana.20029.

12. M. Wolff, A. Brunklaus, S. M. Zuberi, Phenotypic spectrum and genetics of SCN2A-related disorders, treatment options, and outcomes in epilepsy and beyond, *Epilepsia*, 60 Suppl 3 (2019), S59–S67. DOI: https://10.1111/epi.14935.

13. S. M. Zuberi, E. Wirrell, E. Yozawitz, J. M. Wilmshurst, N. Specchio, K. Riney, et al., ILAE classification and definition of epilepsy syndromes with onset in neonates and infants: Position statement by the ILAE Task Force on Nosology and Definitions, *Epilepsia*, 63 (2022), 1349–97. DOI: https://10.1111/epi.17239.

14. E. Herlenius, S. E. Heron, B. E. Grinton, D. Keay, I. E. Scheffer, J. C. Mulley, et al., SCN2A mutations and benign familial neonatal-infantile seizures: The phenotypic spectrum, *Epilepsia*, 48 (2007), 1138–42. DOI: https://0.1111/j.1528-1167.2007.01049.x.

15. C. Reynolds, M. D. King, K. M. Gorman, The phenotypic spectrum of SCN2A-related epilepsy, *Eur J Paediatr Neurol*, 24 (2020), 117–22. DOI: https://10.1016/j.ejpn.2019.12.016.

16. T. T. Sands, M. Balestri, G. Bellini, S. B. Mulkey, O. Danhaive, E. H. Bakken, et al., Rapid and safe response to low-dose carbamazepine in neonatal epilepsy, *Epilepsia*, 57 (2016), 2019–30. DOI: https://10.1111/epi.13596.

17. S. Weckhuysen, A. L. George, Jr., M. R. Cilio, S. James, C. Loewy, T. Sands, et al., *KCNQ2- and KCNQ3-associated epilepsy*, S. Weckhuysen & A. L. George, Jr. (eds.) (Cambridge, UK: Cambridge University Press; 2022).

18. J. H. Döring, A. Saffari, T. Bast, et al., Efficacy, tolerability, and retention of antiseizure medications in PRRT2-associated infantile epilepsy, *Neurol Genet*, 8 (2022), e200020. DOI: https://10.1212/nxg.0000000000200020.

19. J. Lee, Y. O. Kim, B. C. Lim, J. Lee, PRRT2-positive self-limited infantile epilepsy: Initial seizure characteristics and response to sodium channel blockers, *Epilepsia Open*, 8 (2023), 436–43. DOI: https://10.1002/epi4.12708.

20. J. Lee, Y. O. Kim, B. C. Lim, J. Lee, The evolving spectrum of PRRT2-associated paroxysmal diseases, *Brain*, 138 (2015), 3476–95. DOI: https://10.1093/brain/awv317.

21. A. Landolfi, P. Barone, R. Erro, The spectrum of PRRT2-associated disorders: Update on clinical features and pathophysiology, *Front Neurol*, 12 (2021), 629747. DOI: https://10.3389/fneur.2021.629747.

22. R. S. Boerma, K. P. Braun, M. P. van den Broek, F. M. van Berkestijn, M. E. Swinkels, E. O. Hagebeuk, et al., Remarkable phenytoin sensitivity in 4 children with SCN8A-related epilepsy: A molecular neuropharmacological approach, *Neurotherapeutics*, 13 (2016), 192–7. DOI: https://10.1007/s13311-015-0372-8.

23. E. Gardella, F. Becker, R. S. Møller, J. Schubert, J. R. Lemke, L. H. Larsen, et al., Benign infantile seizures and paroxysmal dyskinesia caused by an SCN8A mutation, *Ann Neurol*, 79 (2016), 428–36. DOI: https://10.1002/ana.24580.

24. L. Pons, G. Lesca, D. Sanlaville, N. Chatron, A. Labalme, V. Manel, et al., Neonatal tremor episodes and hyperekplexia-like presentation at onset in a child with SCN8A developmental and epileptic encephalopathy, *Epileptic Disord*, 20 (2018), 289–94. DOI: https://10.1684/epd.2018.0988.

25. J. L. Wagnon, N. E. Mencacci, B. S. Barker, E. R. Wengert, K. P. Bhatia, B. Balint, et al., Partial loss-of-function of sodium channel SCN8A in familial isolated myoclonus, *Hum Mutat*, 39 (2018), 965–9. DOI: https://10.1002/humu.23547.

26. K. M. Johannesen, Y. Liu, M. Koko, C. E. Gjerulfsen, L. Sonnenberg, J. Schubert, et al., Genotype–phenotype correlations in SCN8A-related disorders reveal prognostic and therapeutic implications, *Brain*, 145 (2022), 2991–3009. DOI: https://10.1093/brain/awab321.

27. H. E. Olson, M. Kelly, C. M. LaCoursiere, R. Pinsky, D. Tambunan, C. Shain, et al., Genetics and genotype-phenotype correlations in early onset epileptic encephalopathy with burst suppression, *Ann Neurol*, 81 (2017), 419–29. DOI: https://10.1002/ana.24883.

28. R. Burgess, S. Wang, A. McTague, K. E. Boysen, X. Yang, Q. Zeng, et al., The genetic landscape of epilepsy of infancy with migrating focal seizures, *Ann Neurol*, 86 (2019), 821–31. DOI: https://10.1002/ana.25619.

29. K. B. Howell, J. M. McMahon, G. L. Carvill, D. Tambunan, M. T. Mackay, V. Rodriguez-Casero, et al., SCN2A encephalopathy: A major cause of epilepsy of infancy with migrating focal seizures, *Neurology*, 85 (2015), 958–66. DOI: https://10.1212/wnl.0000000000001926.

30. H. J. Kim, D. Yang, S. H. Kim, B. Kim, H. D. Kim, J. S. Lee, et al., The phenotype and treatment of SCN2A-related developmental and epileptic encephalopathy, *Epileptic Disord*, 22 (2020), 563–70. DOI: https://10.1684/epd.2020.1199.

31. V. Vlachou, L. Larsen, E. Pavlidou, N. Ismayilova, N. D. Mazarakis, M. Pantazi, et al., SCN2A mutation in an infant with Ohtahara syndrome and neuroimaging findings: Expanding the phenotype of neuronal migration disorders, *J Genet*, 98 (2019), 54. DOI: https://10.1007/s12041-019-1104-3.

32. Epilepsy Phenome/Genome Project, Epi4K, Consortium, Diverse genetic causes of polymicrogyria with epilepsy, *Epilepsia*, 62 (2021), 973–83. DOI: https://10.1111/epi.16854.

33. S. K. Akula, A. Y. Chen, J. E. Neil, D. D. Shao, A. Mo, N. K. Hylton, et al., Exome sequencing and the identification of new genes and shared mechanisms in polymicrogyria, *JAMA Neurol*, 80 (2023), 980–8. DOI: https://10.1001/jamaneurol.2023.2363.

34. K. Nakamura, M. Kato, H. Osaka, S. Yamashita, E. Nakagawa, K. Haginoya, et al., Clinical spectrum of SCN2A mutations expanding to Ohtahara syndrome, *Neurology*, 81 (2013), 992–8. DOI: https://10.1212/WNL.0b013e3182a43e57.

35. A. Zerem, D. Lev, L. Blumkin, H. Goldberg-Stern, Y. Michaeli-Yossef, A. Halevy, et al., Paternal germline mosaicism of a SCN2A mutation results in Ohtahara syndrome in half siblings, *Eur J Paediatr Neurol* 18 (2014), 567–71. DOI: https://10.1016/j.ejpn.2014.04.008.

36. S. Ohtahara, Y. Yamatogi, Ohtahara syndrome: With special reference to its developmental aspects for differentiating from early myoclonic encephalopathy, *Epilepsy Research*, 70 Suppl 1 (2006), S58–67. DOI: https://10.1016/j.eplepsyres.2005.11.021.

37. M. Touma, M. Joshi, M. C. Connolly, G. P. Ellen, A. R. Hansen, O. Khwaja, et al., Whole genome sequencing identifies SCN2A mutation in monozygotic twins with Ohtahara syndrome and unique neuropathologic findings, *Epilepsia*, 54 (2013), e81–e5. DOI: https://10.1111/epi.12137.

38. G. Barcia, M. R. Fleming, A. Deligniere, V. R. Gazula, M. R. Brown, M. Langouet, et al., De novo gain-of-function KCNT1 channel mutations cause malignant migrating partial seizures of infancy, *Nat Genet*, 44 (2012), 1255–9. DOI: https://10.1038/ng.2441.

39. C. Ohba, M. Kato, N. Takahashi, H. Osaka, T. Shiihara, J. Tohyama, et al., De novo KCNT1 mutations in early-onset epileptic encephalopathy, *Epilepsia*, 56 (2015), e121–8. DOI: https://10.1111/epi.13072.

40. M. Kato, T. Yamagata, M. Kubota, H. Arai, S. Yamashita, T. Nakagawa, et al., Clinical spectrum of early onset epileptic encephalopathies caused by KCNQ2 mutation, *Epilepsia*, 54 (2013), 1282–7. DOI: https://10.1111/epi.12200.

41. S. J. Sanders, A. J. Campbell, J. R. Cottrell, R. S. Moller, F. F. Wagner, A. L. Auldridge, et al., Progress in understanding and treating SCN2A-mediated disorders, *Trends Neurosci*, 41 (2018), 442–56. DOI: https://10.1016/j.tins.2018.03.011.

42. K. Crawford, J. Xian, K. L. Helbig, P. D. Galer, S. Parthasarathy, D. Lewis-Smith, et al., Computational analysis of 10,860 phenotypic annotations in individuals with SCN2A-related disorders, *Genet Med*, 23 (2021), 1263–72. DOI: https://10.1038/s41436-021-01120-1.

43. D. Samanta, R. Ramakrishnaiah, De novo R853Q mutation of SCN2A gene and West syndrome, *Acta Neurol Belg*, 115 (2015), 773–6. DOI: https://10.1007/s13760-015-0454-8.

44. G. Berecki, K. B. Howell, Y. H. Deerasooriya, M. R. Cilio, M. K. Oliva, D. Kaplan, et al., Dynamic action potential clamp predicts functional separation in mild familial and severe de novo forms of SCN2A epilepsy, *Proc Natl Acad Sci USA*, 115 (2018), E5516–E25. DOI: https://10.1073/pnas.1800077115.

45. A. R. Paciorkowski, L. L. Thio, W. B. Dobyns, Genetic and biologic classification of infantile spasms, *Pediatr Neurol*, 45 (2011), 355–67. DOI: https://10.1016/j.pediatrneurol.2011.08.010.

46. P. Pavone, A. Polizzi, S. D. Marino, G. Corsello, R. Falsaperla, S. Marino, et al., West syndrome: A comprehensive review, *Neurol Sci*, 41 (2020), 3547–62. DOI: https://10.1007/s10072-020-04600-5.

47. N. Chourasia, C. J. Yuskaitis, M. H. Libenson, A. M. Bergin, S. Liu, B. Zhang, et al., Infantile spasms: Assessing the diagnostic yield of an institutional guideline and the impact of etiology on long-term treatment response, *Epilepsia*, 63 (2022), 1164–76. DOI: https://10.1111/epi.17209.

48. R. Richardson, D. Baralle, C. Bennett, T. Briggs, E. K. Bijlsma, J. Clayton-Smith, et al., Further delineation of phenotypic spectrum of SCN2A-related disorder, *Am J Med Genet A*, 188 (2022), 867–77. DOI: https://10.1002/ajmg.a.62595.

49. G. D. Mangano, A. Fontana, V. Antona, V. Salpietro, G. R. Mangano, M. Giuffrè, et al., Commonalities and distinctions between two neurodevelopmental disorder subtypes associated with SCN2A and SCN8A variants and literature review, *Mol Genet Genomic Med*, 10 (2022), e1911. DOI: https://10.1002/mgg3.1911.

50. Y. Liao, A. K. Anttonen, E. Liukkonen, E. Gaily, S. Maljevic, S. Schubert, et al., SCN2A mutation associated with neonatal epilepsy, late-onset episodic ataxia, myoclonus, and pain, *Neurology*, 75 (2010), 1454–8. DOI: https://10.1212/WNL.0b013e3181f8812e.

51. N. Schwarz, A. Hahn, T. Bast, S. Müller, H. Löffler, S. Maljevic, et al., Mutations in the sodium channel gene SCN2A cause neonatal epilepsy with late-onset episodic ataxia, *J Neurol*, 263 (2016), 334–43. DOI: https://10.1007/s00415-015-7984-0.

52. K. M. Gorman, M. D. King, SCN2A p.Ala263Val variant a phenotype of neonatal seizures followed by paroxysmal ataxia in toddlers, *Pediatr Neurol*, 67 (2017), 111–2. DOI: https://10.1016/j.pediatrneurol.2016.11.008.

53. N. Schwarz, T. Bast, E. Gaily, G. Golla, K. M. Gorman, L. R. Griffiths, et al., Clinical and genetic spectrum of SCN2A-associated episodic ataxia, *Eur J Paediatr Neurol*, 23 (2019), 438–47. DOI: https://10.1016/j.ejpn.2019.03.001.

54. E. Amadori, G. Pellino, L. Bansal, S. Mazzone, R. S. Møller, G. Rubboli, et al., Genetic paroxysmal neurological disorders featuring episodic ataxia and epilepsy, *Eur J Med Genet*, 65 (2022), 104450. DOI: https://10.1016/j.ejmg.2022.104450.

55. A. Hackenberg, A. Baumer, H. Sticht, B. Schmitt, J. Kroell-Seger, D. Wille, et al., Infantile epileptic encephalopathy, transient choreoathetotic movements, and hypersomnia due to a de novo missense mutation in the SCN2A gene, *Neuropediatrics*, 45 (2014), 261–4. DOI: https://10.1055/s-0034-1372302.

56. C. Spagnoli, C. Fusco, A. Percesepe, V. Leuzzi, F. Pisani, Genetic neonatal-onset epilepsies and developmental/epileptic encephalopathies with movement disorders: A systematic review, *Int J Mol Sci*, 22 (2021). DOI: https://10.3390/ijms22084202.

57. F. Riant, C. H. Thompson, J. M. DeKeyser, T. V. Abramova, S. Gazal, T. Moulin, et al., Pathogenic SCN2A variants are associated with familial and sporadic hemiplegic migraine, *Research Square* (2023). DOI: https://10.21203/rs.3.rs-3215189/v1.

58. E. Panagiotakaki, F. D. Tiziano, M. A. Mikati, L. S. Vijfhuizen, S. Nicole, G. Lesca, et al., Exome sequencing of ATP1A3-negative cases of alternating hemiplegia of childhood reveals SCN2A as a novel causative gene, *Eur J Hum Genet* 32 (2024), 224–31. DOI: https://10.1038/s41431-023-01489-4.

59. S. Lauxmann, N. E. Verbeek, Y. Liu, M. Zaichuk, S. Müller, J. R. Lemke, et al., Relationship of electrophysiological dysfunction and clinical severity in SCN2A-related epilepsies, *Hum Mutat*, 39 (2018), 1942–56. DOI: https://10.1002/humu.23619

60. A. Brunklaus, R. Ellis, E. Reavey, C. Semsarian, S. M. Zuberi, Genotype phenotype associations across the voltage-gated sodium channel family, *J Med Genet*, 51 (2014), 650–8. DOI: https://10.1136/jmedgenet-2014-102608.

61. Y. Liao, L. Deprez, S. Maljevic, J. Pitsch, L. Claes, D. Hristova, et al., Molecular correlates of age-dependent seizures in an inherited neonatal-infantile epilepsy, *Brain*, 133 (2010), 1403–14. DOI: https://10.1093/brain/awq057.

62. A. Begemann, M. A. Acuña, M. Zweier, M. Vincent, K. Steindl, R. Bachmann-Gagescu, et al., Further corroboration of distinct functional features in SCN2A variants causing intellectual disability or epileptic phenotypes, *Mol Med*, 25 (2019), 6. DOI: https://10.1186/s10020-019-0073-6.

63. C. H. Thompson, F. Potet, T. V. Abramova, J. M. DeKeyser, N. F. Ghabra, C. G. Vanoye, et al., Epilepsy-associated SCN2A (Na$_V$1.2) variants exhibit diverse and complex functional properties, *J Gen Physiol*, 155 (2023), e202313375. DOI: https://10.1085/jgp.202313375.

64. S. Syrbe, B. S. Zhorov, A. Bertsche, M. K. Bernhard, F. Hornemann, U. Mütze, et al., Phenotypic variability from benign infantile epilepsy to Ohtahara syndrome associated with a novel mutation in SCN2A, *Mol Syndromol*, 7 (2016), 182–8. DOI: https://10.1159/000447526.

65. A. L. Baasch, I. Hüning, C. Gilissen, J. Klepper, J. A. Veltman, G. Gillessen-Kaesbach, et al., Exome sequencing identifies a de novo SCN2A mutation in a patient with intractable seizures, severe intellectual disability, optic atrophy, muscular hypotonia, and brain abnormalities, *Epilepsia*, 55 (2014), e25–9. DOI: https://10.1111/epi.12554.

66. G. Berecki, K. B. Howell, J. Heighway, N. Olivier, J. Rodda, I. Overmars, et al., Functional correlates of clinical phenotype and severity in recurrent SCN2A variants, *Commun Biol*, 5 (2022), 515. DOI: https://10.1038/s42003-022-03454-1.

67. K. M. Johannesen, M. J. Miranda, H. Lerche, R. S. Møller, Letter to the editor: Confirming neonatal seizure and late onset ataxia in SCN2A Ala263Val, *J Neurol*, 263 (2016), 1459–60. DOI: https://10.1007/s00415-016-8149-5.

68. R. Ben-Shalom, C. M. Keeshen, K. N. Berrios, J. Y. An, S. J. Sanders, K. J. Bender, Opposing effects on Na$_V$1.2 function underlie differences between SCN2A variants observed in individuals with autism spectrum disorder or infantile seizures, *Biol Psychiatry*, 82 (2017), 224–32. DOI: https://10.1016/j.biopsych.2017.01.009.

69. S. Richards, N. Aziz, S. Bale, D. Bick, S. Das, J. Gastier-Foster, et al., Standards and guidelines for the interpretation of sequence variants: A joint consensus recommendation of the American College of Medical Genetics and Genomics and the Association for Molecular Pathology, *Genet Med*, 17 (2015), 405–24. DOI: https://10.1038/gim.2015.30.

70. T. Brandt, L. M. Sack, D. Arjona, D. Tan, H. Mei, H. Cui, et al., Adapting ACMG/AMP sequence variant classification guidelines for single-gene copy number variants, *Genet Med*, 22 (2020), 336–44. DOI: https://10.1038/s41436-019-0655-2.

71. E. R. Riggs, E. F. Andersen, A. M. Cherry, S. Kantarci, H. Kearney, A. Patel, et al., Technical standards for the interpretation and reporting of constitutional copy-number variants: A joint consensus recommendation of the American College of Medical Genetics and Genomics (ACMG) and the Clinical Genome Resource (ClinGen), *Genet Med*, 22 (2020), 245–57. DOI: https://10.1038/s41436-019-0686-8.

72. M. Noda, T. Ikeda, T. Kayano, H. Suzuki, H. Takeshima, M. Kurasaki, et al., Existence of distinct sodium channel messenger RNAs in rat brain, *Nature*, 320 (1986), 188–92. DOI: https://10.1038/320188a0.

73. M. Noda, T. Ikeda, T. Suzuki, H. Takeshima, T. Takahashi, M. Kuno, et al., Expression of functional sodium channels from cloned cDNA, *Nature*, 322 (1986), 826–8. DOI: https://10.1038/322826a0.

74. C. M. I. Ahmed, D. H. Ware, S. C. Lee, C. D. Patten, A. V. Ferrer-Montiel, A. F. Schinder, et al., Primary structure, chromosomal localization, and functional expression of a voltage-gated sodium channel from human brain, *Proc Natl Acad Sci U S A*, 89 (1992), 8220–4. DOI: https://10.1073/pnas.89.17.8220.

75. M. Noda, S. Shimizu, T. Tanabe, T. Takai, T. Kayano, T. Ikeda, et al., Primary structure of *Electrophorus electricus* sodium channel deduced from cDNA sequence, *Nature*, 312 (1984), 121–7. DOI: https://10.1038/312121a0.

76. S. H. Heinemann, H. Terlau, W. Stühmer, K. Imoto, S. Numa, Calcium channel characteristics conferred on the sodium channel by single mutations, *Nature*, 356 (1992), 441–3. DOI: https://10.1038/356441a0.

77. T. Schlief, R. Schönherr, K. Imoto, S. H. Heinemann, Pore properties of rat brain II sodium channels mutated in the selectivity filter domain, *Eur Biophys J*, 25 (1996), 75–91. DOI: https://10.1007/s0024900 50020.

78. W. Stühmer, F. Conti, H. Suzuki, X. D. Wang, M. Noda, N. Yahagi, et al., Structural parts involved in activation and inactivation of the sodium channel, *Nature*, 339 (1989), 597–603. DOI: https://10.1038/339597a0.

79. H. K. Motoike, H. Liu, I. W. Glaaser, A. S. Yang, M. Tateyama, R. S. Kass, The Na^{+} channel inactivation gate is a molecular complex: A novel role of the COOH-terminal domain, *J Gen Physiol*, 123 (2004), 155–65. DOI: https://10.1085/jgp.200308929.

80. D. L. Capes, M. P. Goldschen-Ohm, M. Arcisio-Miranda, F. Bezanilla, B. Chanda, Domain IV voltage-sensor movement is both sufficient and rate limiting for fast inactivation in sodium channels, *J Gen Physiol*, 142 (2013), 101–12. DOI: https://10.1085/jgp.201310998.

81. W. A. Catterall, Voltage-gated sodium channels at 60: Structure, function and pathophysiology, *J Physiol*, 590 (2012), 2577–89. DOI: https://10.1113/jphysiol.2011.224204.

82. W. A. Catterall, G. Wisedchaisri, N. Zheng, The chemical basis for electrical signaling, *Nat Chem Biol*, 13 (2017), 455–63. DOI: https://10.1038/nchembio.2353.

83. W. A. Catterall, M. J. Lenaeus, T. M. Gamal El-Din, Structure and pharmacology of voltage-gated sodium and calcium channels, *Annu Rev Pharmacol Toxicol*, 60 (2020), 133–54. DOI: https://10.1146/annurev-pharmtox-010818-021757.

84. X. Pan, Z. Li, X. Huang, G. Huang, S. Gao, H. Shen, et al., Molecular basis for pore blockade of human Na^+ channel $Na_V1.2$ by the μ-conotoxin KIIIA, *Science*, 363 (2019), 1309–13. DOI: https://10.1126/science.aaw2999.

85. B. P. Bean, The action potential in mammalian central neurons, *Nat Rev Neurosci*, 8 (2007), 451–65. DOI: https://10.1038/nrn2148.

86. G. Stuart, B. Sakmann, Amplification of EPSPs by axosomatic sodium channels in neocortical pyramidal neurons, *Neuron*, 15 (1995), 1065–76. DOI: https://10.1016/0896-6273(95)90095-0.

87. G. Stuart, Voltage-activated sodium channels amplify inhibition in neocortical pyramidal neurons, *Nat Neurosci*, 2 (1999), 144–50. DOI: https://10.1038/5698.

88. J. Yamada-Hanff, B. P. Bean, Persistent sodium current drives conditional pacemaking in CA1 pyramidal neurons under muscarinic stimulation, *J Neurosci*, 33 (2013), 15011–21. DOI: https://10.1523/jneurosci.0577-13.2013.

89. R. Sarao, S. K. Gupta, V. J. Auld, R. J. Dunn, Developmentally regulated alternative RNA splicing of rat brain sodium channel mRNAs, *Nucleic Acids Res*, 19 (1991), 5673–9. DOI: https://10.1093/nar/19.20.5673.

90. P. J. Yarowsky, B. K. Krueger, C. E. Olson, E. C. Clevinger, R. D. Koos, Brain and heart sodium channel subtype mRNA expression in rat cerebral cortex, *Proc Natl Acad Sci U S A*, 88 (1991), 9453–7. DOI: https://10.1073/pnas.88.21.9453.

91. C. H. Thompson, R. Ben-Shalom, K. J. Bender, A. L. George Jr., Alternative splicing potentiates dysfunction of early onset epileptic encephalopathy SCN2A variants, *J Gen Physiol*, 152 (2020), e201912442. DOI: https://10.1085/jgp.201912442.

92. L. Liang, S. Fazel Darbandi, S. Pochareddy, F. O. Gulden, M. C. Gilson, B. K. Sheppard, et al., Developmental dynamics of voltage-gated sodium channel isoform expression in the human and mouse brain, *Genome Med*, 13 (2021), 135. DOI: https://10.1186/s13073-021-00949-0.

93. J. Heighway, A. Sedo, A. Garg, L. Eldershaw, V. Perreau, G. Berecki, et al., Sodium channel expression and transcript variation in the developing brain of human, Rhesus monkey, and mouse, *Neurobiol Dis*, 164 (2022), 105622. DOI: https://10.1016/j.nbd.2022.105622.

94. R. Xu, E. A. Thomas, M. Jenkins, E. V. Gazina, C. Chiu, S. E. Heron, et al., A childhood epilepsy mutation reveals a role for developmentally regulated splicing of a sodium channel, *Mol Cell Neurosci*, 35 (2007), 292–301. DOI: https://10.1016/j.mcn.2007.03.003.

95. E. V. Gazina, B. T. Leaw, K. L. Richards, V. C. Wimmer, T. H. Kim, T. D. Aumann, et al., "Neonatal" $Na_V1.2$ reduces neuronal excitability and affects seizure susceptibility and behaviour, *Hum Mol Genet*, 24 (2015), 1457–68. DOI: https://10.1093/hmg/ddu562.

96. L. L. Isom, K. S. De Jongh, D. E. Patton, B. F. X. Reber, J. Offord, H. Charbonneau, et al., Primary structure and functional expression of the ß1 subunit of the rat brain sodium channel, *Science*, 256 (1992), 839–42. DOI: https://10.1126/science.1375395.

97. L. L. Isom, D. S. Ragsdale, K. S. De Jongh, R. E. Westenbroek, B. F. X. Reber, T. Scheuer, et al., Structure and function of the ß2 subunit of brain sodium channels, a transmembrane glycoprotein with a CAM motif, *Cell*, 83 (1995), 433–42. DOI: https://10.1016/0092-8674(95) 90121-3.

98. J. D. Calhoun, L. L. Isom, The role of non-pore-forming β subunits in physiology and pathophysiology of voltage-gated sodium channels, *Handb Exp Pharmacol*, 221 (2014), 51–89. DOI: https://10.1007/978-3-642-41588-3_4.

99. A. M. Rush, E. K. Wittmack, L. Tyrrell, J. A. Black, S. D. Dib-Hajj, S. G. Waxman, Differential modulation of sodium channel $Na_V1.6$ by two members of the fibroblast growth factor homologous factor 2 subfamily, *Eur J Neurosci*, 23 (2006), 2551–62. DOI: https://10.1111/j.1460-9568.2006.04789.x.

100. F. Laezza, A. Lampert, M. A. Kozel, B. R. Gerber, A. M. Rush, J. M. Nerbonne, et al., FGF14 N-terminal splice variants differentially modulate $Na_V1.2$ and $Na_V1.6$-encoded sodium channels, *Mol Cell Neurosci*, 42 (2009), 90–101. DOI: https://10.1016/j.mcn.2009.05.007.

101. C. H. Thompson, N. A. Hawkins, J. A. Kearney, A. L. George Jr., CaMKII modulates sodium current in neurons from epileptic Scn2a mutant mice,

Proc Natl Acad Sci USA, 114 (2017), 1696–701. DOI: https://10.1073/pnas.1615774114.

102. C. Wang, B. C. Chung, H. Yan, H. G. Wang, S. Y. Lee, G. S. Pitt, Structural analyses of Ca^{2+}/CaM interaction with Na_V channel C-termini reveal mechanisms of calcium-dependent regulation, *Nat Commun*, 5 (2014), 4896. DOI: https://10.1038/ncomms5896.

103. A. D. Nelson, A. M. Catalfio, J. M. Gupta, L. Min, R. N. Caballero-Floran, K. P. Dean, et al., Physical and functional convergence of the autism risk genes *Scn2a* and *Ank2* in neocortical pyramidal cell dendrites, *Neuron* 112 (2024): 1133–49.e6. https://10.1016/j.neuron.2024.01.003.

104. J. P. Gupta, P. M. Jenkins, Ankyrin-B is lipid-modified by S-palmitoylation to promote dendritic membrane scaffolding of voltage-gated sodium channel $Na_V1.2$ in neurons, *Front Physiol*, 14 (2023), 959660. DOI: https://10.3389/fphys.2023.959660.

105. W. Hu, C. Tian, T. Li, M. Yang, H. Hou, Y. Shu, Distinct contributions of $Na_V1.6$ and $Na_V1.2$ in action potential initiation and backpropagation, *Nat Neurosci*, 12 (2009), 996–1002. DOI: https://10.1038/nn.2359.

106. T. Li, C. Tian, P. Scalmani, C. Frassoni, M. Mantegazza, Y. Wang, et al., Action potential initiation in neocortical inhibitory interneurons, *PLoS Biol*, 12 (2014), e1001944. DOI: https://10.1371/journal.pbio.1001944.

107. C. Tian, K. Wang, W. Ke, H. Guo, Y. Shu, Molecular identity of axonal sodium channels in human cortical pyramidal cells, *Front Cell Neurosci*, 8 (2014), 297. DOI: https://10.3389/fncel.2014.00297.

108. T. Yamagata, I. Ogiwara, E. Mazaki, Y. Yanagawa, K. Yamakawa, $Na_V1.2$ is expressed in caudal ganglionic eminence-derived disinhibitory interneurons: Mutually exclusive distributions of $Na_V1.1$ and $Na_V1.2$, *Biochem Biophys Res Commun*, 491 (2017), 1070–6. DOI: https://10.1016/j.bbrc.2017.08.013.

109. T. Yamagata, I. Ogiwara, T. Tatsukawa, T. Suzuki, Y. Otsuka, N. Imaeda, et al., Scn1a-GFP transgenic mouse revealed $Na_V1.1$ expression in neocortical pyramidal tract projection neurons, *Elife*, 12 (2023). DOI: https://10.7554/eLife.87495.

110. J. Yang, Y. Xiao, L. Li, Q. He, M. Li, Y. Shu, Biophysical properties of somatic and axonal voltage-gated sodium channels in midbrain dopaminergic neurons, *Front Cell Neurosci*, 13 (2019), 317. DOI: https://10.3389/fncel.2019.00317.

111. R. Yamano, H. Miyazaki, N. Nukina, The diffuse distribution of $Na_V1.2$ on mid-axonal regions is a marker for unmyelinated fibers in the central nervous system, *Neurosci Res*, 177 (2022), 145–50. DOI: https://10.1016/j.neures.2021.11.005.

112. P. W. E. Spratt, R. Ben-Shalom, C. M. Keeshen, K. J. Burke, Jr., R. L. Clarkson, S. J. Sanders, et al., The autism-associated gene Scn2a contributes to dendritic excitability and synaptic function in the prefrontal cortex, *Neuron*, 103 (2019), 673–85. DOI: https://10.1016/j.neuron.2019.05.037.

113. P. W. E. Spratt, R. P. D. Alexander, R. Ben-Shalom, A. Sahagun, H. Kyoung, C. M. Keeshen, et al., Paradoxical hyperexcitability from Na$_V$1.2 sodium channel loss in neocortical pyramidal cells, *Cell Rep*, 36 (2021), 109483. DOI: https://10.1016/j.celrep.2021.109483.

114. K. M. Goff, E. M. Goldberg, Vasoactive intestinal peptide-expressing interneurons are impaired in a mouse model of Dravet syndrome, *Elife*, 8 (2019), e46846. DOI: https://10.7554/eLife.46846.

115. K. J. Bender, L. O. Trussell, The physiology of the axon initial segment, *Annu Rev Neurosci*, 35 (2012), 249–65. DOI: https://10.1146/annurev-neuro-062111-150339.

116. M. Ye, J. Yang, C. Tian, Q. Zhu, L. Yin, S. Jiang, et al., Differential roles of Na$_V$1.2 and Na$_V$1.6 in regulating neuronal excitability at febrile temperature and distinct contributions to febrile seizures, *Sci Rep*, 8 (2018), 753. DOI: https://10.1038/s41598-017-17344-8.

117. H. Miyazaki, F. Oyama, R. Inoue, T. Aosaki, T. Abe, H. Kiyonari, et al., Singular localization of sodium channel β4 subunit in unmyelinated fibres and its role in the striatum, *Nat Commun*, 5 (2014), 5525. DOI: https://10.1038/ncomms6525.

118. W. Wang, S. Takashima, Y. Segawa, M. Itoh, X. Shi, S. K. Hwang, et al., The developmental changes of Na$_V$1.1 and Na$_V$1.2 expression in the human hippocampus and temporal lobe, *Brain Res*, 1389 (2011), 61–70. DOI: https://10.1016/j.brainres.2011.02.083.

119. W. Shin, H. Kweon, R. Kang, D. Kim, K. Kim, M. Kang, et al., Scn2a haploinsufficiency in mice suppresses hippocampal neuronal excitability, excitatory synaptic drive, and long-term potentiation, and spatial learning and memory, *Front Mol Neurosci*, 12 (2019), 145. DOI: https://10.3389/fnmol.2019.00145.

120. C. Wang, K. D. Derderian, E. Hamada, X. Zhou, A. D. Nelson, H. Kyoung, et al., Impaired cerebellar plasticity hypersensitizes sensory reflexes in SCN2A-associated ASD, *Neuron* 112 (2024), 1444–1455. https://10.1016/j.neuron.2024.01.029.

121. H. O. Heyne, D. Baez-Nieto, S. Iqbal, D. S. Palmer, A. Brunklaus, P. May, et al., Predicting functional effects of missense variants in voltage-gated sodium and calcium channels, *Sci Transl Med*, 12 (2020), eaay6848. DOI: https://10.1126/scitranslmed.aay6848.

122. A. Brunklaus, A. L. George, Jr., D. Lal, E. L. Heinzen, A. M. Goldman, Prophecy or empiricism? Clinical value of predicting versus determining genetic variant functions, *Epilepsia*, 64 (2023), 2909–13. DOI: https://10.1111/epi.17743.

123. R. Ben-Shalom, A. Ladd, N. S. Artherya, C. Cross, K. G. Kim, H. Sanghevi, et al., NeuroGPU: Accelerating multi-compartment, biophysically detailed neuron simulations on GPUs, *J Neurosci Methods*, 366 (2022), 109400. DOI: https://10.1016/j.jneumeth.2021.109400.

124. K. A. Kruth, T. M. Grisolano, C. A. Ahern, A. J. Williams, SCN2A channelopathies in the autism spectrum of neuropsychiatric disorders: a role for pluripotent stem cells? *Molecular Autism*, 11 (2020), 23. DOI: https://10.1186/s13229-020-00330-9.

125. D. Simkin, C. Ambrosi, K. A. Marshall, L. A. Williams, J. Eisenberg, M. Gharib, et al., "Channeling" therapeutic discovery for epileptic encephalopathy through iPSC technologies, *Trends Pharmacol Sci*, 43 (2022), 392–405. DOI: https://10.1016/j.tips.2022.03.001.

126. Z. Que, M. I. Olivero-Acosta, J. Zhang, M. Eaton, A. M. Tukker, X. Chen, et al., Hyperexcitability and pharmacological responsiveness of cortical neurons derived from human iPSCs carrying epilepsy-associated sodium channel $Na_V1.2$-L1342P genetic variant, *J Neurosci*, 41 (2021), 10194–208. DOI: https://10.1523/jneurosci.0564-21.2021.

127. R. Asadollahi, I. Delvendahl, R. Muff, G. Tan, D. G. Rodríguez, S. Turan, et al., Pathogenic SCN2A variants cause early-stage dysfunction in patient-derived neurons, *Hum Mol Genet*, 32 (2023), 2192–204. DOI: https://10.1093/hmg/ddad048.

128. M. Mao, C. Mattei, B. Rollo, S. Byars, C. Cuddy, G. Berecki, et al., Distinctive in vitro phenotypes in iPSC-derived neurons from patients with gain- and loss-of-function *SCN2A* developmental and epileptic encephalopathy, *J Neurosci*, 44 (2024), e0692232023. https://10.1523/JNEUROSCI.0692-23.2023.

129. I. Ogiwara, K. Ito, Y. Sawaishi, H. Osaka, E. Mazaki, I. Inoue, et al., De novo mutations of voltage-gated sodium channel αII gene SCN2A in intractable epilepsies, *Neurology*, 73 (2009), 1046–53. DOI: https://10.1212/WNL.0b013e3181b9cebc.

130. X. Shi, S. Yasumoto, E. Nakagawa, T. Fukasawa, S. Uchiya, S. Hirose, Missense mutation of the sodium channel gene SCN2A causes Dravet syndrome, *Brain Dev*, 31 (2009), 758–62. DOI: https://10.1016/j.braindev.2009.08.009.

131. J. A. Kearney, N. W. Plummer, M. R. Smith, J. Kapur, T. R. Cummins, S. G. Waxman, et al., A gain-of-function mutation in the sodium channel

gene Scn2a results in seizures and behavioral abnormalities, *Neuroscience*, 102 (2001), 307–17. DOI: https://10.1016/s0306-4522 (00)00479-6.

132. S. K. Bergren, S. Chen, A. Galecki, J. A. Kearney, Genetic modifiers affecting severity of epilepsy caused by mutation of sodium channel Scn2a, *Mamm Genome*, 16 (2005), 683–90. DOI: https://10.1007/s00335-005-0049-4.

133. B. S. Jorge, C. M. Campbell, A. R. Miller, E. D. Rutter, C. A. Gurnett, C. G. Vanoye, et al., Voltage-gated potassium channel KCNV2 ($K_V8.2$) contributes to epilepsy susceptibility, *Proc Natl Acad Sci USA*, 108 (2011), 5443–8. DOI: https://10.1073/pnas.1017539108.

134. N. A. Hawkins, J. A. Kearney, Confirmation of an epilepsy modifier locus on mouse chromosome 11 and candidate gene analysis by RNA-Seq, *Genes Brain Behav*, 11 (2012), 452–60. DOI: https://10.1111/j.1601-183X.2012.00790.x.

135. J. D. Calhoun, N. A. Hawkins, N. J. Zachwieja, J. A. Kearney, Cacna1g is a genetic modifier of epilepsy caused by mutation of voltage-gated sodium channel Scn2a, *Epilepsia*, 57 (2016), e103–e7. DOI: https://10.1111/epi.13811.

136. M. Li, N. Jancovski, P. Jafar-Nejad, L. E. Burbano, B. Rollo, K. Richards, et al., Antisense oligonucleotide therapy reduces seizures and extends life span in an SCN2A gain-of-function epilepsy model, *J Clin Invest*, 131 (2021), e152079. DOI: https://10.1172/JCI152079.

137. L. Jia, *A platform for analysis of in vitro neuronal networks for the development of precision therapeutics in SCN2A disease* (Melbourne, Australia: University of Melbourne, 2019).

138. D. M. Echevarria-Cooper, N. A. Hawkins, S. N. Misra, A. M. Huffman, T. Thaxton, C. H. Thompson, et al., Cellular and behavioral effects of altered $Na_V1.2$ sodium channel ion permeability in *Scn2a* K1422E mice, *Hum Mol Genet*, 31 (2022), 2964–88. DOI: https://10.1093/hmg/ddac087.

139. S. K. Sundaram, H. T. Chugani, V. N. Tiwari, A. H. M. M. Huq, SCN2A mutation is associated with infantile spasms and bitemporal glucose hypometabolism, *Ped Neurol*, 49 (2013), 46–9. DOI: https://10.1016/j.pediatrneurol.2013.03.002.

140. D. M. Echevarria-Cooper, N. A. Hawkins, J. A. Kearney, Strain-dependent effects on neurobehavioral and seizure phenotypes in Scn2a (K1422E) mice, *bioRxiv* (2023). DOI: https://10.1101/2023.06.06.543929.

141. D. M. Echevarria-Cooper, J. A. Kearney, Evaluating the interplay between estrous cyclicity and flurothyl-induced seizure susceptibility in Scn2a

(K1422E) mice, *MicroPubl Biol*, 2023 (2023). DOI: https://10.17912/micropub.biology.000850.

142. S. J. Sanders, M. T. Murtha, A. R. Gupta, J. D. Murdoch, M. J. Raubeson, A. J. Willsey, et al., De novo mutations revealed by whole-exome sequencing are strongly associated with autism, *Nature*, 485 (2012), 237–41. DOI: https://10.1038/nature10945.

143. F. K. Satterstrom, J. A. Kosmicki, J. Wang, et al., Large-scale exome sequencing study implicates both developmental and functional changes in the neurobiology of autism, *Cell*, 180 (2020), 568–84.e23. DOI: https://10.1016/j.cell.2019.12.036.

144. J. M. Fu, F. K. Satterstrom, M. Peng, H. Brand, R. L. Collins, S. Dong, et al., Rare coding variation provides insight into the genetic architecture and phenotypic context of autism, *Nat Genet*, 54 (2022), 1320–31. DOI: https://10.1038/s41588-022-01104-0.

145. H. Hu, P. Jonas, A supercritical density of Na_+ channels ensures fast signaling in GABAergic interneuron axons, *Nat Neurosci*, 17 (2014), 686–93. DOI: https://10.1038/nn.3678.

146. S. J. Middleton, E. M. Kneller, S. Chen, I. Ogiwara, M. Montal, K. Yamakawa, et al., Altered hippocampal replay is associated with memory impairment in mice heterozygous for the Scn2a gene, *Nat Neurosci*, 21 (2018), 996–1003. DOI: https://10.1038/s41593-018-0163-8.

147. M. R. Carey, Synaptic mechanisms of sensorimotor learning in the cerebellum, *Curr Opin Neurobiol*, 21 (2011), 609–15. DOI: https://10.1016/j.conb.2011.06.011.

148. J. D. Schmahmann, The cerebellum and cognition, *Neurosci Lett*, 688 (2019), 62–75. DOI: https://10.1016/j.neulet.2018.07.005.

149. R. Planells-Cases, M. Caprini, J. Zhang, E. M. Rockenstein, R. R. Rivera, C. Murre, et al., Neuronal death and perinatal lethality in voltage-gated sodium channel alpha(II)-deficient mice, *Biophys J*, 78 (2000), 2878–91. DOI: https://10.1016/s0006-3495(00)76829-9.

150. J. Zhang, X. Chen, M. Eaton, J. Wu, Z. Ma, S. Lai, et al., Severe deficiency of the voltage-gated sodium channel $Na_V1.2$ elevates neuronal excitability in adult mice, *Cell Rep*, 36 (2021), 109495. DOI: https://10.1016/j.celrep.2021.109495.

151. Z. Ma, M. Eaton, Y. Liu, J. Zhang, X. Chen, X. Tu, et al., Deficiency of autism-related Scn2a gene in mice disrupts sleep patterns and circadian rhythms, *Neurobiol Dis*, 168 (2022), 105690. DOI: https://10.1016/j.nbd.2022.105690.

152. M. Eaton, J. Zhang, Z. Ma, A. C. Park, E. Lietzke, C. M. Romero, et al., Generation and basic characterization of a gene-trap knockout mouse

model of Scn2a with a substantial reduction of voltage-gated sodium channel $Na_V1.2$ expression, *Genes Brain Behav*, 20 (2021), e12725. DOI: https://10.1111/gbb.12725.

153. I. Ogiwara, H. Miyamoto, T. Tatsukawa, T. Yamagata, T. Nakayama, N. Atapour, et al., $Na_V1.2$ haplodeficiency in excitatory neurons causes absence-like seizures in mice, *Commun Biol*, 1 (2018), 96. DOI: https://10.1038/s42003-018-0099-2.

154. K. B. Howell, J. M. McMahon, G. L. Carvill, D. Tambunan, M. T. Mackay, V. Rodriguez-Casero, et al., *SCN2A* encephalopathy: A major cause of epilepsy of infancy with migrating focal seizures, *Neurology*, 85 (2015), 958–66. DOI: https://10.1212/WNL.0000000000001926.

155. J. B. O'Connor, E. B. Kirschenblatt, L. Laux, A. T. Berg, S. N. Misra, J. J. Millichap, Seizure semiology and response to treatment in a pediatric cohort with SCN2A variants: A parent report, *medRxiv* (2023), 2023.02.23.23286378. DOI: https://10.1101/2023.02.23.23286378.

156. R. Dilena, P. Striano, E. Gennaro, et al., Efficacy of sodium channel blockers in SCN2A early infantile epileptic encephalopathy, *Brain Dev*, 39 (2017), 345–8. DOI: https://10.1016/j.braindev.2016.10.015.

157. T. Welzel, V. C. Ziesenitz, S. Waldvogel, S. Scheidegger, P. Weber, J. N. van den Anker, et al., Use of a personalized phenytoin dosing approach to manage difficult to control seizures in an infant with a SCN2A mutation, *Eur J Clin Pharmacol*, 75 (2019), 737–9. DOI: https://10.1007/s00228-019-02629-w.

158. J. H. Karnes, A. E. Rettie, A. A. Somogyi, R. Huddart, A. E. Fohner, C. M. Formea, et al., Clinical Pharmacogenetics Implementation Consortium (CPIC) guideline for CYP2C9 and HLA-B genotypes and phenytoin dosing: 2020 update, *Clin Pharmacol Ther*, 109 (2021), 302–9. DOI: https://10.1002/cpt.2008.

159. S. K. Adney, J. J. Millichap, J. M. DeKeyser, T. Abramova, C. H. Thompson, A. L. George Jr. , Functional and pharmacological evaluation of a novel SCN2A variant linked to early-onset epilepsy, *Ann Clin Transl Neurol*, 79 (2020), 1488–1501. DOI: https://10.1002/acn3.51105.

160. L. L. Anderson, C. H. Thompson, N. A. Hawkins, R. D. Nath, A. A. Petersohn, S. Rajamani, et al., Antiepileptic activity of preferential inhibitors of persistent sodium current, *Epilepsia*, 55 (2014), 1274–83. DOI: https://10.1111/epi.12657.

161. S. Fredj, K. J. Sampson, H. Liu, R. S. Kass, Molecular basis of ranolazine block of LQT-3 mutant sodium channels: Evidence for site of action, *Br J Pharmacol*, 148 (2006), 16–24. DOI: https://10.1038/sj.bjp.0706709.

162. K. M. Kahlig, I. Lepist, K. Leung, S. Rajamani, A. L. George Jr., Ranolazine selectively blocks persistent current evoked by epilepsy-associated $Na_V1.1$ mutations, *Br J Pharmacol*, 161 (2010), 1414–26. DOI: https://10.1111/j.1476-5381.2010.00976.x.

163. K. M. Kahlig, R. Hirakawa, L. Liu, A. L. George, Jr., L. Belardinelli, S. Rajamani, Ranolazine reduces neuronal excitability by interacting with inactivated states of brain sodium channels, *Mol Pharmacol*, 85 (2014), 162–74. DOI: https://10.1124/mol.113.088492.

164. D. O. Koltun, E. Q. Parkhill, E. Elzein, T. Kobayashi, G. T. Notte, R. Kalla, et al., Discovery of triazolopyridine GS-458967, a late sodium current inhibitor (Late INai) of the cardiac $Na_V1.5$ channel with improved efficacy and potency relative to ranolazine, *Bioorg Med Chem Lett*, 26 (2016), 3202–6. DOI: https://10.1016/j.bmcl.2016.03.101.

165. E. R. Mason, T. R. Cummins, Differential inhibition of human Nav1.2 resurgent and persistent sodium currents by cannabidiol and GS967, *Int J Mol Sci*, 21 (2020). DOI: https://10.3390/ijms21072454.

166. E. M. Baker, C. H. Thompson, N. A. Hawkins, J. L. Wagnon, E. R. Wengert, M. K. Patel, et al., The novel sodium channel modulator GS-458967 (GS967) is an effective treatment in a mouse model of SCN8A encephalopathy, *Epilepsia*, 59 (2018), 1166–76. DOI: https://10.1111/epi.14196.

167. E. R. Wengert, A. U. Saga, P. S. Panchal, B. S. Barker, M. K. Patel, Prax330 reduces persistent and resurgent sodium channel currents and neuronal hyperexcitability of subiculum neurons in a mouse model of SCN8A epileptic encephalopathy, *Neuropharmacology*, 158 (2019), 107699. DOI: https://10.1016/j.neuropharm.2019.107699.

168. F. Potet, C. G. Vanoye, A. L. George Jr., Use-dependent block of human cardiac sodium channels by GS967, *Mol Pharm*, 90 (2016), 52–6. DOI: https://10.1124/mol.116.103358/.

169. K. M. Kahlig, L. Scott, R. J. Hatch, A. Griffin, G. Martinez Botella, Z. A. Hughes, et al., The novel persistent sodium current inhibitor PRAX-562 has potent anticonvulsant activity with improved protective index relative to standard of care sodium channel blockers, *Epilepsia*, 63 (2022), 697–708. DOI: https://10.1111/epi.17149.

170. J. P. Johnson, T. Focken, K. Khakh, P. K. Tari, C. Dube, S. J. Goodchild, et al., NBI-921352, a first-in-class, $Na_V1.6$ selective, sodium channel inhibitor that prevents seizures in Scn8a gain-of-function mice, and

wild-type mice and rats, *Elife*, 11 (2022), e72468. DOI: https://10.7554/eLife.72468.

171. R. Mahalingam, M. Oldham, C. Puryear, P. Bansal, B. Sriram, D. Patel, et al., PRAX-562–102: A phase 1 trial evaluating the safety, tolerability, pharmacokinetics and pharmacodynamics of PRAX-562 in healthy volunteers (P4-9.011), *Neurology*, 100 (2023), 3192. DOI: https://10.1212/wnl.0000000000203090.

172. R. S. Finkel, E. Mercuri, B. T. Darras, A. M. Connolly, N. L. Kuntz, J. Kirschner, et al., Nusinersen versus sham control in infantile-onset spinal muscular atrophy, *N Engl J Med*, 377 (2017), 1723–32. DOI: https://10.1056/NEJMoa1702752.

173. E. Mercuri, B. T. Darras, C. A. Chiriboga, J. W. Day, C. Campbell, A. M. Connolly, et al., Nusinersen versus sham control in later-onset spinal muscular atrophy, *N Engl J Med*, 378 (2018), 625–35. DOI: https://10.1056/NEJMoa1710504.

174. S. T. Crooke, X. H. Liang, B. F. Baker, R. M. Crooke, Antisense technology: A review, *J Biol Chem*, 296 (2021), 100416. DOI: https://10.1016/j.jbc.2021.100416.

175. G. L. Carvill, T. Matheny, J. Hesselberth, S. Demarest, Haploinsufficiency, dominant negative, and gain-of-function mechanisms in epilepsy: Matching therapeutic approach to the pathophysiology, *Neurotherapeutics*, 18 (2021), 1500–14. DOI: https://10.1007/s13311-021-01137-z.

176. S. F. Hill, M. H. Meisler, Antisense oligonucleotide therapy for neurodevelopmental disorders, *Dev Neurosci*, 43 (2021), 247–52. DOI: https://10.1159/000517686.

177. C. F. Bennett, H. B. Kordasiewicz, D. W. Cleveland, Antisense drugs make sense for neurological diseases, *Annu Rev Pharmacol Toxicol*, 61 (2021), 831–52. DOI: https://10.1146/annurev-pharmtox-010919-023738.

178. M. E. McCauley, C. F. Bennett, Antisense drugs for rare and ultra-rare genetic neurological diseases, *Neuron*, 111 (2023), 2465–8. DOI: https://10.1016/j.neuron.2023.05.027.

179. D. Ta, J. Downs, G. Baynam, A. Wilson, P. Richmond, H. Leonard, A brief history of MECP2 duplication syndrome: 20-years of clinical understanding, *Orphanet J Rare Dis*, 17 (2022), 131. DOI: https://10.1186/s13023-022-02278-w.

180. M. A. Mortberg, J. E. Gentile, N. Nadaf, C. Vanderburg, S. Simmons, D. Dubinsky, et al., A single-cell map of antisense oligonucleotide activity in the brain, *Nucleic Acids Res*, 51 (2023). 7109–24. https://10.1093/nar/gkad371

181. N. D. Germain, W. K. Chung, P. D. Sarmiere, RNA interference (RNAi)-based therapeutics for treatment of rare neurologic diseases, *Mol Aspects Med*, 91 (2023), 101148. DOI: https://10.1016/j.mam.2022 .101148.

182. L. Bendixen, T. I. Jensen, R. O. Bak, CRISPR-Cas-mediated transcriptional modulation: The therapeutic promises of CRISPRa and CRISPRi, *Mol Ther*, 31 (2023), 1920–37. DOI: https://10.1016/j.ymthe.2023.03.024.

183. J. C. Carpenter, G. Lignani, Gene editing and modulation: The Holy Grail for the genetic epilepsies? *Neurotherapeutics*, 18 (2021), 1515–23. DOI: https://10.1007/s13311-021-01081-y.

184. E. M. Porto, A. C. Komor, I. M. Slaymaker, G. W. Yeo, Base editing: Advances and therapeutic opportunities, *Nat Rev Drug Discov*, 19 (2020), 839–59. DOI: https://10.1038/s41573-020-0084-6.

185. P. J. Chen, D. R. Liu, Prime editing for precise and highly versatile genome manipulation, *Nat Rev Genet*, 24 (2023), 161–77. DOI: https:// 10.1038/s41576-022-00541-1.

186. J. R. Davis, S. Banskota, J. M. Levy, G. A. Newby, X. Wang, A. V. Anzalone, et al., Efficient prime editing in mouse brain, liver and heart with dual AAVs, *Nat Biotechnol*, 42 (2023)253–64. DOI: https:// 10.1038/s41587-023-01758-z.

187. S. Tamura, A. D. Nelson, P. W. E. Spratt, H. Kyoung, X. Zhou, Z. Li, et al., CRISPR activation rescues abnormalities in *SCN2A* haploinsufficiency-associated autism spectrum disorder, *bioRxiv* (2022), 2022.03.30.486483. DOI: https://10.1101/2022.03.30.486483.

188. G. Colasante, G. Lignani, S. Brusco, C. Di Berardino, J. Carpenter, S. Giannelli, et al., dCas9-based Scn1a gene activation restores inhibitory interneuron excitability and attenuates seizures in Dravet syndrome mice, *Mol Ther*, 28 (2020), 235–53. DOI: https://10.1016/j.ymthe.2019.08.018.

189. A. Tanenhaus, T. Stowe, A. Young, J. McLaughlin, R. Aeran, I. W. Lin, et al., Cell-selective adeno-associated virus-mediated SCN1A gene regulation therapy rescues mortality and seizure phenotypes in a Dravet syndrome mouse model and is well tolerated in nonhuman primates, *Hum Gene Ther*, 33 (2022), 579–97. DOI: https://10.1089/hum.2022.037.

190. G. L. Carvill, H. C. Mefford, Poison exons in neurodevelopment and disease, *Curr Opin Genet Dev*, 65 (2020), 98–102. DOI: https://10.1016/ j.gde.2020.05.030.

191. Z. Han, C. Chen, A. Christiansen, S. Ji, Q. Lin, C. Anumonwo, et al., Antisense oligonucleotides increase Scn1a expression and reduce seizures and SUDEP incidence in a mouse model of Dravet syndrome, *Sci Transl Med*, 12 (2020), eaaz6100. DOI: https://10.1126/scitranslmed.aaz6100.

192. E. R. Wengert, P. K. Wagley, S. M. Strohm, N. Reza, I. C. Wenker, R. P. Gaykema, et al., Targeted augmentation of nuclear gene output (TANGO) of Scn1a rescues parvalbumin interneuron excitability and reduces seizures in a mouse model of Dravet Syndrome, *Brain Res*, 1775 (2022), 147743. DOI: https://10.1016/j.brainres.2021.147743.

193. S. Fadila, B. Beucher, I. G. Dopeso-Reyes, A. Mavashov, M. Brusel, K. Anderson, et al., Viral vector-mediated expression of $Na_V1.1$, after seizure onset, reduces epilepsy in mice with Dravet syndrome, *J Clin Invest*, 133 (2023), e159316. DOI: https://10.1172/jci159316.

194. L. Mora-Jimenez, M. Valencia, R. Sanchez-Carpintero, J. Tønnesen, S. Fadila, M. Rubinstein, et al., Transfer of SCN1A to the brain of adolescent mouse model of Dravet syndrome improves epileptic, motor, and behavioral manifestations, *Mol Ther Nucleic Acids*, 25 (2021), 585–602. DOI: https://10.1016/j.omtn.2021.08.003.

195. E. Chilcott, J. A. Díaz, C. Bertram, M. Berti, R. Karda, Genetic therapeutic advancements for Dravet syndrome, *Epilepsy Behav*, 132 (2022), 108741. DOI: https://10.1016/j.yebeh.2022.108741.

196. J. D. Lueck, J. S. Yoon, A. Perales-Puchalt, A. L. Mackey, D. T. Infield, M. A. Behlke, et al., Engineered transfer RNAs for suppression of premature termination codons, *Nat Commun*, 10 (2019), 822. DOI: https://10.1038/s41467-019-08329-4.

197. J. J. Porter, C. S. Heil, J. D. Lueck, Therapeutic promise of engineered nonsense suppressor tRNAs, *Wiley Interdiscip Rev RNA*, 12 (2021), e1641. DOI: https://10.1002/wrna.1641.

198. J. Wang, Y. Zhang, C. A. Mendonca, O. Yukselen, K. Muneeruddin, L. Ren, et al., AAV-delivered suppressor tRNA overcomes a nonsense mutation in mice, *Nature*, 604 (2022), 343–8. DOI: https://10.1038/s41586-022-04533-3.

199. E. Dolgin, tRNA therapeutics burst onto startup scene, *Nat Biotechnol*, 40 (2022), 283–6. DOI: https://10.1038/s41587-022-01252-y.

200. C. A. Ahern, *A tRNA-based gene therapy approach for high-fidelity repair of SCN2A premature termination codons* (New York: Simons Foundation Autism Research Initiative, 2019).

201. D. C. Brock, S. Demarest, T. A. Benke, Clinical trial design for disease-modifying therapies for genetic epilepsies, *Neurotherapeutics*, 18 (2021), 1445–57. DOI: https://10.1007/s13311-021-01123-5.

202. M. Strupp, R. Kalla, J. Claassen, C. Adrion, U. Mansmann, T. Klopstock, et al., A randomized trial of 4-aminopyridine in EA2 and related familial episodic ataxias, *Neurology*, 77 (2011), 269–75. DOI: https://10.1212/WNL.0b013e318225ab07.

203. A. T. Berg, H. Palac, G. Wilkening, F. Zelko, L. Schust Meyer, SCN2A-developmental and epileptic encephalopathies: Challenges to trial-readiness for non-seizure outcomes, *Epilepsia*, 62 (2021), 258–68. DOI: https://10.1111/epi.16750.

204. A. S. Allen, S. F. Berkovic, P. Cossette, N. Delanty, D. Dlugos, E. E. Eichler, et al., De novo mutations in epileptic encephalopathies, *Nature*, 501 (2013), 217–21. DOI: https://10.1038/nature12439.

205. Y. Kobayashi, J. Tohyama, M. Kato, N. Akasaka, S. Magara, H. Kawashima, et al., High prevalence of genetic alterations in early-onset epileptic encephalopathies associated with infantile movement disorders, *Brain Dev*, 38 (2016), 285–92. DOI: https://10.1016/j.braindev.2015.09.011.

206. Y. Kong, K. Yan, L. Hu, M. Wang, X. Dong, Y. Lu, et al., Data on mutations and clinical features in SCN1A or SCN2A gene, *Data Brief*, 22 (2019), 492–501. DOI: https://10.1016/j.dib.2018.08.122.

207. S. Vidal, N. Brandi, P. Pacheco, J. Maynou, G. Fernandez, C. Xiol, et al., The most recurrent monogenic disorders that overlap with the phenotype of Rett syndrome, *Eur J Paediatr Neurol*, 23 (2019), 609–20. DOI: https://10.1016/j.ejpn.2019.04.006.

208. E. Chérot, B. Keren, C. Dubourg, W. Carré, M. Fradin, A. Lavillaureix, et al., Using medical exome sequencing to identify the causes of neuro-developmental disorders: Experience of 2 clinical units and 216 patients, *Clin Genet*, 93 (2018), 567–76. DOI: https://10.1111/cge.13102.

209. S. Ganguly, C. H. Thompson, A. L. George Jr., Enhanced slow inactivation contributes to dysfunction of a recurrent SCN2A mutation associated with developmental and epileptic encephalopathy, *J Physiol*, 599 (2021), 4375–88. DOI: https://10.1113/jp281834.

210. S. B. Linley, M. M. Gallo, R. P. Vertes, Lesions of the ventral midline thalamus produce deficits in reversal learning and attention on an odor texture set shifting task, *Brain Res*, 1649 (2016), 110–22. DOI: https://10.1016/j.brainres.2016.08.022.

211. E. Parrini, C. Marini, D. Mei, A. Galuppi, E. Cellini, D. Pucatti, et al., Diagnostic targeted resequencing in 349 patients with drug-resistant pediatric epilepsies identifies causative mutations in 30 different genes, *Hum Mutat*, 38 (2017), 216–25. DOI: https://10.1002/humu.23149.

212. M. Nashabat, X. S. Al Qahtani, S. Almakdob, W. Altwaijri, D. M. Ba-Armah, K. Hundallah, et al., The landscape of early infantile epileptic encephalopathy in a consanguineous population, *Seizure*, 69 (2019), 154–72. DOI: https://10.1016/j.seizure.2019.04.018.

213. N. Trump, A. McTague, H. Brittain, A. Papandreou, E. Meyer, A. Ngoh, et al., Improving diagnosis and broadening the phenotypes in early-onset

seizure and severe developmental delay disorders through gene panel analysis, *J Med Genet*, 53 (2016), 310–7. DOI: https://10.1136/jmed genet-2015-103263.

214. E. R. Mason, F. Wu, R. R. Patel, Y. Xiao, S. C. Cannon, T. R. Cummins, Resurgent and gating pore currents induced by de novo *SCN2A* epilepsy mutations, *eNeuro*, 6 (2019), ENEURO.0141-19.2019. DOI: https://10.1523/eneuro.0141-19.2019.

215. N. M. Allen, J. Conroy, A. Shahwan, B. Lynch, R. G. Correa, S. D. Pena, et al., Unexplained early onset epileptic encephalopathy: Exome screening and phenotype expansion, *Epilepsia*, 57 (2016), e12–7. DOI: https://10.1111/epi.13250.

216. P. Miao, J. Feng, Y. Guo, J. Wang, X. Xu, Y. Wang, et al., Genotype and phenotype analysis using an epilepsy-associated gene panel in Chinese pediatric epilepsy patients, *Clin Genet*, 94 (2018), 512–20. DOI: https://10.1111/cge.13441.

217. P. Miao, S. Tang, J. Ye, J. Wang, Y. Lou, B. Zhang, et al., Electrophysiological features: The next precise step for SCN2A developmental epileptic encephalopathy, *Mol Genet Genomic Med*, 8 (2020), e1250. DOI: https://10.1002/mgg3.1250.

218. D. Matalon, E. Goldberg, L. Medne, E. D. Marsh, Confirming an expanded spectrum of SCN2A mutations: a case series, *Epileptic Disord*, 16 (2014), 13–8. DOI: https://10.1684/epd.2014.0641.

219. S. Dimassi, A. Labalme, D. Ville, A. Calender, C. Mignot, N. Boutry-Kryza, et al., Whole-exome sequencing improves the diagnosis yield in sporadic infantile spasm syndrome, *Clin Genet*, 89 (2016), 198–204. DOI: https://10.1111/cge.12636.

220. S. N. Misra, K. M. Kahlig, A. L. George Jr., Impaired Na$_V$1.2 function and reduced cell surface expression in benign familial neonatal-infantile seizures, *Epilepsia*, 49 (2008), 1535–45. DOI: https://10.1111/j.1528-1167.2008.01619.x.

221. W. Fazeli, K. Becker, P. Herkenrath, C. Düchting, F. Körber, P. Landgraf, et al., Dominant SCN2A mutation causes familial episodic ataxia and impairment of speech development, *Neuropediatrics*, 49 (2018), 379–84. DOI: https://10.1055/s-0038-1668141.

222. S. Gokben, H. Onay, S. Yilmaz, T. Atik, G. Serdaroglu, H. Tekin, et al., Targeted next generation sequencing: the diagnostic value in early-onset epileptic encephalopathy, *Acta Neurol Belg*, 117 (2017), 131–8. DOI: https://10.1007/s13760-016-0709-z.

223. T. U. J. Bruun, C. L. DesRoches, D. Wilson, V. Chau, T. Nakagawa, M. Yamasaki, et al., Prospective cohort study for identification of

underlying genetic causes in neonatal encephalopathy using whole-exome sequencing, *Genet Med*, 20 (2018), 486–94. DOI: https://10.1038/gim.2017.129.

224. Q. Zhang, J. Li, Y. Zhao, X. Bao, L. Wei, J. Wang, Gene mutation analysis of 175 Chinese patients with early-onset epileptic encephalopathy, *Clin Genet*, 91 (2017), 717–24. DOI: https://10.1111/cge.12901.

Acknowledgments

We are grateful to Louise M. Tiranoff, PhD, Founder and Managing Director of Tiranoff Productions and GeneticaLens, who produced Video 3 with the editing assistance of Adam DeSantes. We acknowledge Adil Wafa for creating Figure 9, and Shaye Moore for proofreading the manuscript and transcribing the videos.

About the Authors

Alfred L. George, Jr., M.D. is Professor and Chair of Pharmacology at Northwestern University Feinberg School of Medicine. He has been a pioneer in elucidating the genetics and pathogenesis of channelopathies with a focus on genetic disorders caused by voltage-gated ion channel mutations including KCNQ2-associated epilepsy. He was the director of the Channelopathy-Associated Epilepsy Research Center without Walls funded by the National Institute of Neurological Disorders and Stroke.

Megan Abbott, M.D. is a pediatric neurologist at Children's Hospital Colorado with clinical and research interests in neurogenetic conditions within epilepsy. In summer 2024, she became an assistant professor at the University of Colorado in the Department of Pediatrics, Division of Neurology. Her research is specifically looking at outcome measures that can be generalized across many developmental and epileptic encephalopathies including *SCN2A*.

Kevin J. Bender, Ph.D. is a Professor of Neurology at the University of California, San Francisco. He is a leader in studying the mechanisms by which neurons integrate information, and how these processes are disrupted in neuropsychiatric and neurodevelopmental disorders, including SCN2A-related disorders.

Andreas Brunklaus, M.D. is a consultant paediatric neurologist at the Royal Hospital for Children, Glasgow and honorary professor at the University of Glasgow. He is an international expert in sodium channel disorders including *SCN2A*-related disorders and leads international research collaborations developing diagnostic tools in epilepsy genetics.

Scott Demarest, M.D., M.S.C.S. is an Associate Professor in the Department of Pediatrics, Division of Neurology at the University of Colorado. His clinical practice and research focus on the evaluation and treatment of neurogenetic epilepsies including clinical trials for novel therapeutics, natural history studies and the development of improved outcome measures. He is the Clinical Director of Precision Medicine Institute at Children's Hospital Colorado where he supports diagnostic and therapeutic approaches to improve patient outcomes.

Shawn Egan, Ph.D. is a parent of a child affected by an SCN2A-related disorder, and he serves as Chief Scientific Officer for the FamilieSCN2A Foundation. In this role, Shawn focuses on building the necessary infrastructure to expedite the development of treatments and cures for all patients with SCN2A-related disorders. This includes empowering the SCN2A community and providing support for SCN2A-related research and drug development.

Isabel Haviland, M.D. is a research fellow in neurology at Boston Children's Hospital and Harvard Medical School. She is focused on clinical research exploring genotype-phenotype correlations in pediatric genetic epilepsies.

Jennifer A. Kearney, Ph.D. is an Associate Professor of Pharmacology at Northwestern University Feinberg School of Medicine, the Center for Genetic Medicine and the Center for Autism and Neurodevelopment. Her research program is focused on identifying genetic factors that contribute to childhood epilepsies and neurodevelopmental disorders. Her research has contributed to understanding the genetic basis and impact of genetic modifiers on SCN2A-realted disorders using genetically engineered mouse models.

Leah Schust Myers, M.S. is the founder and Executive Director for the FamilieSCN2A Foundation. She has spent her entire career working in health care administration and never imagined she would find a use for her skills in an entirely different way. From medical secretary to hospital manager and everywhere in between, Leah learned how to manage the needs of large populations within a medical setting. When her son was diagnosed with an SCN2A-related disorder in 2012, it became abundantly clear how to leverage her experience to help others.

Heather E. Olson, M.D. is an Assistant Professor in the Department of Neurology, Division of Epilepsy and Clinical Neurophysiology at Boston Children's Hospital. She is a pediatric neurologist with expertise in epilepsy genetics and fetal/neonatal neurology. She directs a clinical research program focusing on early-onset genetic developmental and epileptic encephalopathies, including CDKL5 Deficiency Disorder and SCN2A-related disorders.

Stephan J. Sanders, BMBS, Ph.D. is a Professor of Paediatric Neurogenetics at the University of Oxford and Associate Professor at the University of California, San Francisco. He leads a group that identifies the genetic causes of neurodevelopmental disorders and seeks to understand the consequent neurobiology and identify genome-targeted therapies. His research demonstrated that *de novo SCN2A* mutations are associated with autism spectrum disorders and the differing phenotypes of gain- and loss-of function variants.

Christina SanInocencio, Ph.D. is an Assistant Professor of communication at Fairfield University and adjunct professor of health communication at Stony Brook University. She has been a leader in rare epilepsy advocacy for nearly two decades and serves as a member of TASCO (team for advancing science and clinical outcomes) for FamilieSCN2A Foundation.

Joseph Symonds, M.B., Ch.B., Ph.D. is a Senior Clinical Research Fellow at the School of Health & Wellbeing at the University of Glasgow. He is a Consultant Paediatric Neurologist at the Royal Hospital for Children, Glasgow where is delivers epilepsy care for children and young people and runs a genetic epilepsy clinic. His research takes an epidemiological approach to understanding the frequency of rare genetic epilepsies, and defining the true phenotypic spectrum of each genetic epilepsy.

Christopher H. Thompson, Ph.D. is a Research Assistant Professor of Pharmacology at Northwestern Feinberg School of Medicine. His work has contributed to the elucidation of functional consequences of pathogenic variants associated with SCN2A-associated neurodevelopmental disorders, as well as pharmacology and regulation of voltage-gated sodium channels.

Cambridge Elements ≡

Genetics in Epilepsy

Annapurna H. Poduri

Boston Children's Hospital and Harvard Medical School

Annapurna H. Poduri, MD, MPH is Associate Professor of Neurology at Harvard Medical School. She is Director of the Epilepsy Genetics Program at Boston Children's Hospital, which focuses on the discovery of germline and mosaic variants in patients with epilepsy, and modeling epilepsy genes in zebrafish and cell-based models.

Alfred L. George, Jr.

Northwestern University Feinberg School of Medicine

Alfred L. George, Jr., MD, is Professor and Chair of Pharmacology at the Northwestern University Feinberg School of Medicine. He directs the Channelopathy-associated Epilepsy Research Center without Walls, supported by the National Institutes of Neurological Disorders and Stroke, connecting patient variants with bench science.

Erin L. Heinzen

University of North Carolina, Chapel Hill

Erin L. Heinzen, PharmD, PhD, is Associate Professor of Pharmacy and Genetics at the University of North Carolina at Chapel Hill. She has served as Principal Investigator of the Sequencing, Biostatistics and Bioinformatics Core of the Epi4 K Consortium and investigates somatic mosaic mutation in epilepsy and the mechanisms underlying SLC35A2 epilepsy.

Associate Editor

Sara James

KCNQ2 Cure Alliance and Genetic Epilepsy Team Australia

Sara James is a renowned broadcast journalist and an advocate for research in epilepsy and community–academic partnerships in genetic epilepsy. She is Vice President of the KCNQ2 Cure Alliance and a co-founder of Genetic Epilepsy Team Australia.

About the Series

Recent advances in epilepsy genetics are actively revealing numerous genetic contributors to epilepsy, both inherited and noninherited, collectively accounting for a substantial portion of otherwise unexplained epilepsies. This series integrates clinical epilepsy genetics and laboratory research, driving the field towards more precise and effective treatments.

Cambridge Elements $^{\equiv}$

Genetics in Epilepsy

Printed in the United States
by Baker & Taylor Publisher Services